PHOTOGRAPHY
by NAZLI DEVELI

DESIGN
by STUDIO AURORA

EDITOR
STELLA NILSSON

Hardcover Edition - Revised & Expanded Second Printing, February 2022
ISBN 9781736374269
Independently published by Nazlı Develi

For information about permission to reproduce selections
from this book, write to hello@gurmevegan.com
www.gurmevegan.com
www.greenandawake.com

GREEN & AWAKE

GOURMET RAW

140 VIBRANT LIVING FOOD RECIPES

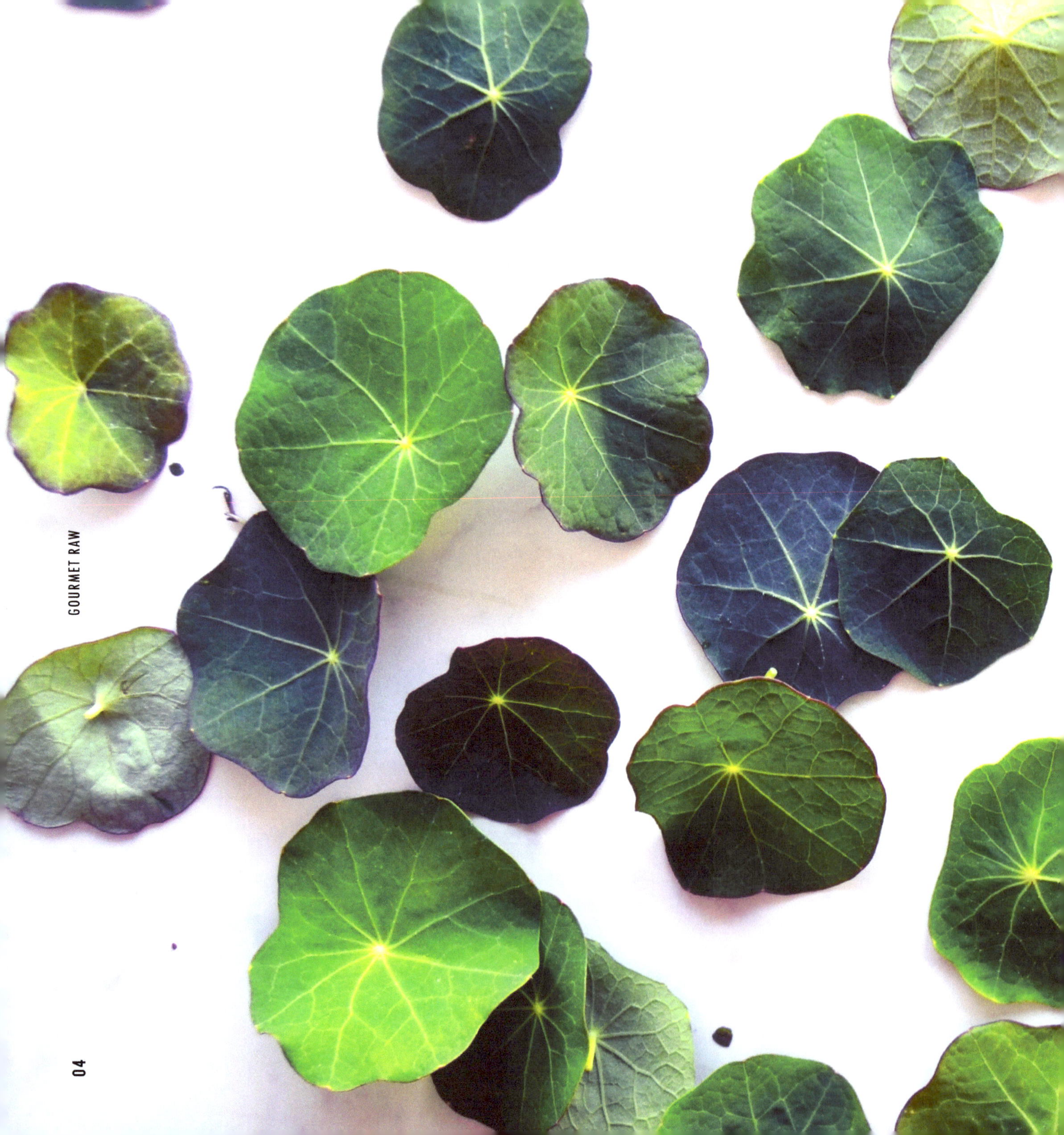

CONTENT

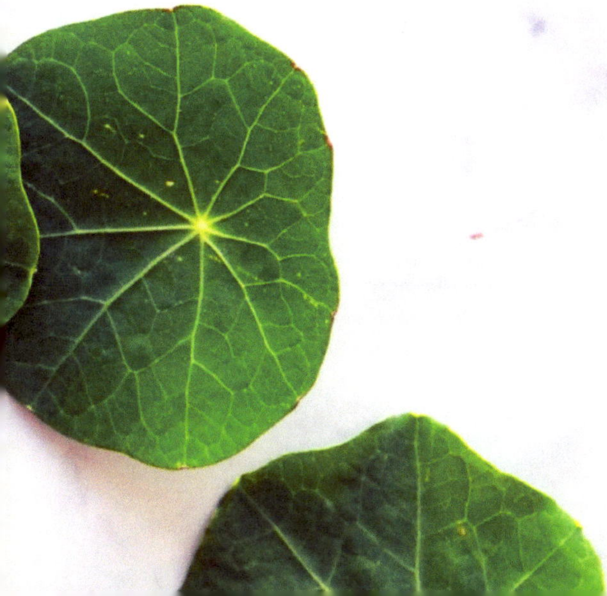

STIMULATE

RIGHT BRAIN

THROUGH LIVING FOOD

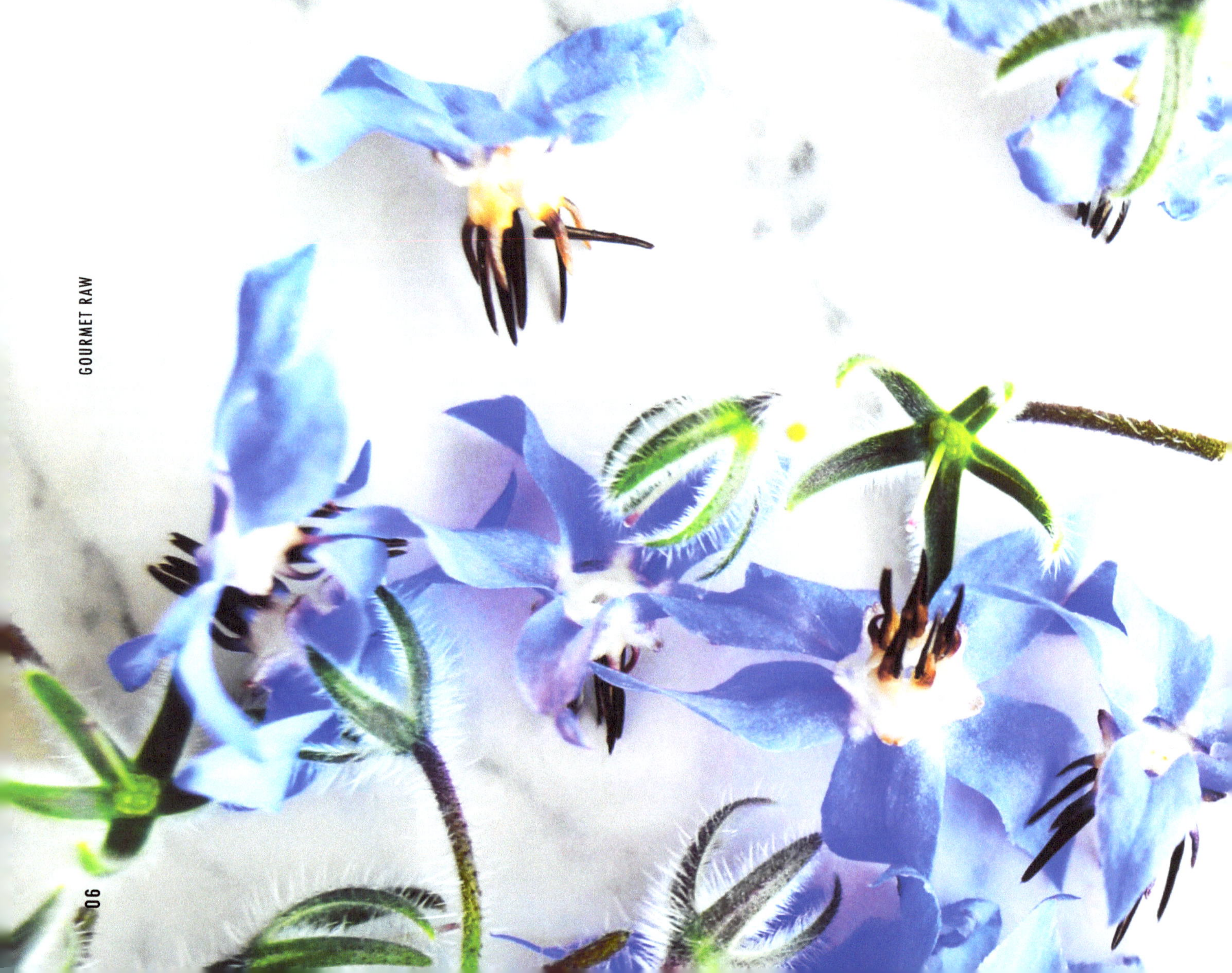

KEYS TO RAW FOOD

WHY 42° C?

Living food is a powerful natural healing force, which gradually restores the microelectrical potential and overall functioning of every cell in our body. The basic premise behind of raw food is that cooking and processing foods decreases their digestibility and vitamin, mineral density as well as their overall health-promoting qualities. We dehydrate everything under 42°Celcius because when we heat food above 42°C (107°Fahrenheit) the enzyme content is destroyed. Enzymes are necessary for almost every function in body especially digestion.

SOAKING & SPROUTING

Phytic acid is a compound found in all legumes, grains, and nuts. This compound is known to inhibit the absorption of crucial minerals and nutrients in the body. By soaking and sprouting all legumes, grains, and nuts we reduce the amount of phytic acid. We eat legumes and grains after soaking, sprouting or dehydrating. Nuts are also good protein sources but they are acidic. When we soak them before using to activate enyzme inhibitors, we will be cleaned them and they will be ready to eat safe.

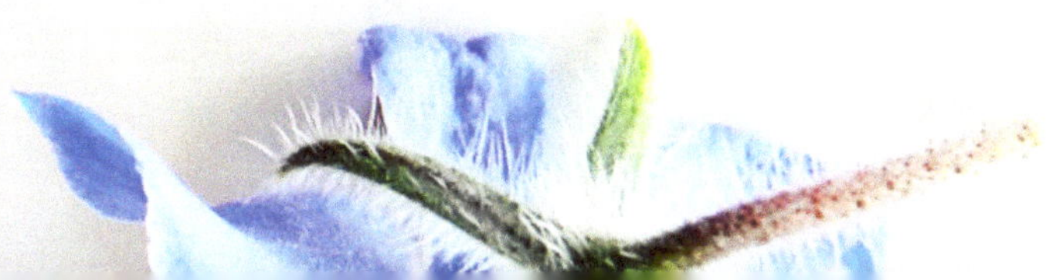

RAW ACTIVATION

There's one thing I'm pretty sure of, there's a tape recorder inside us. It is within us even though we can't always get there. We water ourselves through experiences, thoughts and food in this three dimensonal physical world and we get it's results. So it is very important to eat right, act ethical, work on beneficial works, and bring solutions instead complains by finding our life purpose. The feeling of doing good can make you feel happy and fulfilled with your life.

Years ago, transition to veganism was just a step for me. I would say that it changed me incredibly, but something was missing. As a person who always questions, I started to think that why are vegan dishes are an imitation of animal food. I wonder if our body needs to take such intense gluten from processed foods like seitan.

RE-LEARNING TASTES & HEALTH

Most of us don't like brussels sprouts or broccoli, when we boil it , all its nutritional value dies. We do not know that we should eat raw, this is not taught to us. Whereas they taste better when consumed raw. Humans, domesticated pets and farm animals are the only species that eat cooked food. They are also the only get degenerative diseases. You can not see a wild animal in the forest coming down with diseases like cancer.
Remember that highly processed cooked food were introduced into markets in the 1930's and the statistics show meteoric rises in cancer rates since that decade.
Eating cooked, processed (any kind of packaged food) is a fruitless way of feeding ourselves. Because food enyzmes have been destroyed, our body has to use its own enyzmes to digest to cooked food. So, the enyzme preservation is the key to longevity.

ENERGY ACTIVATION

Cooked food also has lack of biophotons. Every living organism emits biophotons.
Living foods contain the biophoton light energy for your body. It is thought that the higher the level of light energy a cell emits, the greater its vitality and the potential for the transfer of that energy to the individual who consumes it. The more light a food is able to store, the more nutritious it is. Naturally grown fresh raw vegetables, for example, and sun-ripened fresh fruits, are rich in light energy. The capacity to store biophotons is therefore a measure of the quality of your food.

RIGHT BRAIN ACTIVATION

I believe that our daily food choices are some of the most impactful choices we make when it comes to spiritual awarness.

Our inner genius lies in the right side of the brain. To try to access this part of the brain, we can undergone sleep deprivation experiments, drink Ayahuasca, go fruit-based diet, fasting and breathing practices to experience what life is like when the left-hand side falls asleep and the right side takes over. But the safest way is to experience this by returning to a balanced fruit-based raw diet by supporting breathing practices.

Unfortunately our brains are became damaged over thousands of years by eating an incorrect diet. Most of us don't know this, but when you dare to experience, I know it is hard to leave comfort zone for most people but, I can say that you will find yourself in a different world.
The most significant change for me is to feel like I am getting younger everyday.
I also met with many people like me, those eat raw food, have the highest energy, clarity of mind, neurotransmitter production and joy in life .

KEEPING THE BALANCE

Our left brain hemisphere is responsible for tasks we think as more male-orianted; linear, rational, logical. The left one is independent thinker, the ego which understands itself as separate from the rest of the world, an isolated part. European culture is left brain dominant. Some of us may have developed our right hemispheres more than others but most of us are ruled by the left brain. We are tend to protect our lives in this materialist world in order to live a safe life. People need to keep controlling theirselves and this requires left brain function.

Today we live in a world with endless wars that is leading by people who are left-brain dominated. In order to achieve enlightment and to recover our natural state of bliss, we must learn to balance the two hemispheres.

To stimulate right brain, we should consume more raw food. Creative pursuits, painting, drawing, using left hand, meditation, yoga, book writing, all helps building new pathways in the brain which create a grater state of balance. As we move more into our right brains, we literally learn new ways of thinking and this allow to discover the true potential of human consciousness. We begin to consider what is good for the whole in an upcoming situation; not just what will purely benefit to ourselves.of this irritation, the plaques can either choke off the artery or rupture their pus filled contents into the blood stream which contributes to arterial damage and results in the heart attack.

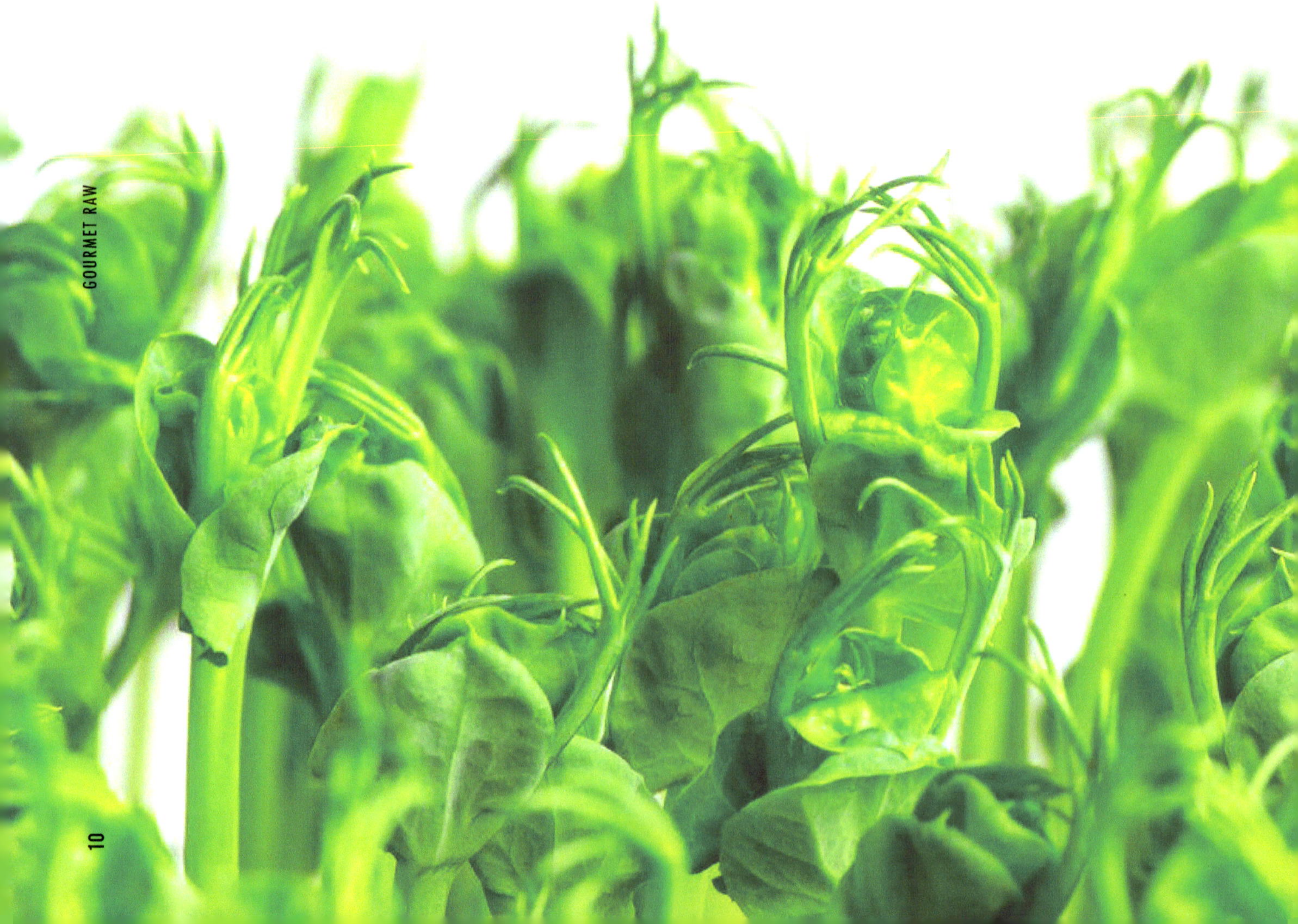

"GOURMET RAW" brings a creative twist to raw foods in a fun and artistic way with flavor infusions that will rock your taste buds .

If you think "raw food" means zucchini noodles or just salad, "Raw" will astound you with it's elegance and inventiveness. It's a combination raw cookbook, featuring gourmet recipes using raw and dehydrated vegetables, sprouted whole grains, legumes, nuts and fruits.

In this book some recipes are very easy to make but some recipes are not quick to prepare, and many include references to other recipes.
It is for those who want to add some fancy raw plates to their restaurant menu or just want to try new things in their kitchen.

With so many overcomplicated aspects of our lives, it's refreshing to pare down and create simple raw meals that are still bursting with flavor!

Thank you for buying this book and I hope you will enjoy as much as I do.

GOURMET RAW

Food Designer, Chef & Author

"RAW FOOD IS A PORTAL TO HIGHER DIMENSIONS"

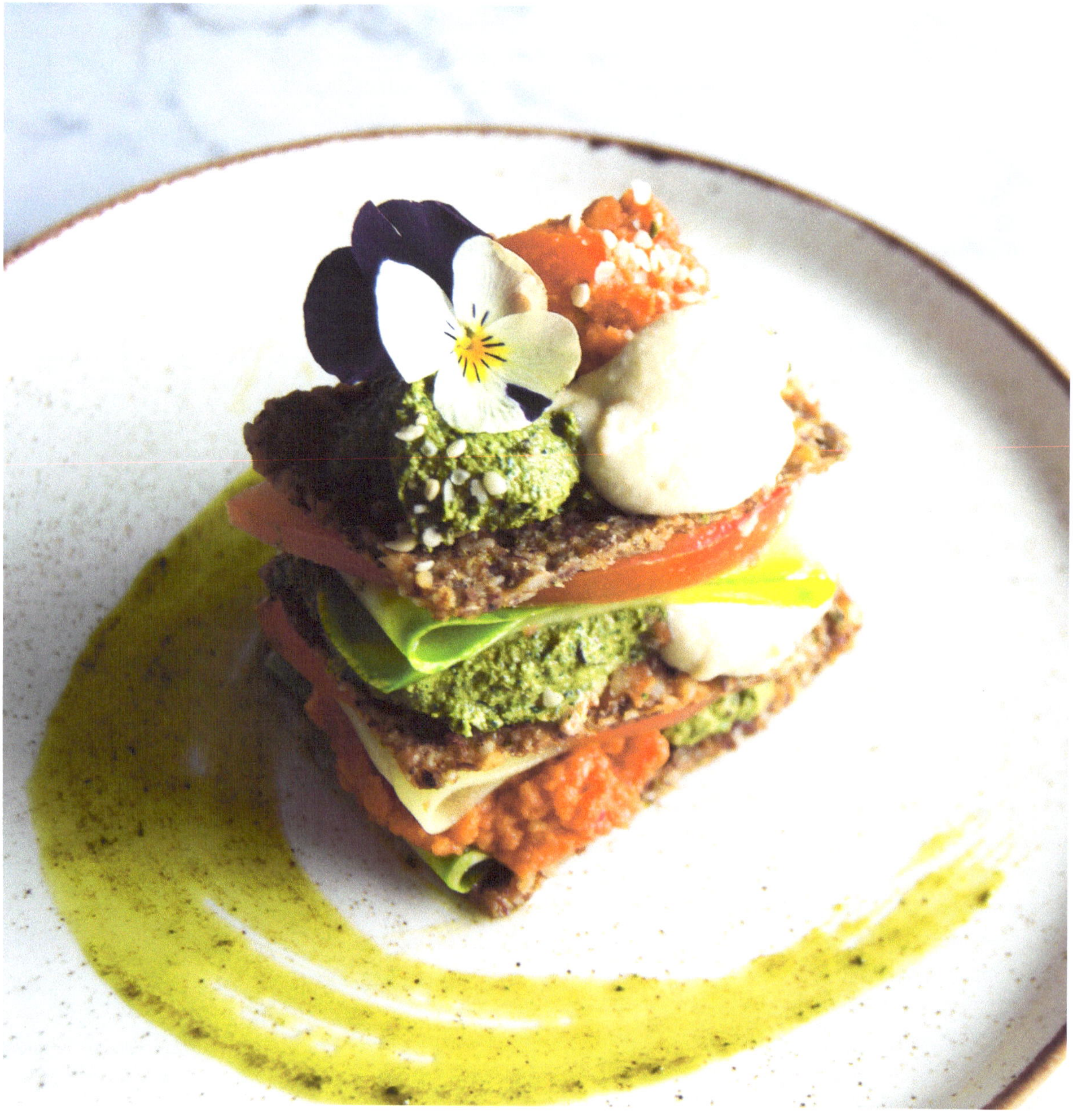

QUEEN LASAGNA

Yield: 2-3 person

Base
2 medium zucchini
1 large heirloom tomato
8-9 slices raw flat bread
Hemp hearts to serve
Pink himalayan salt to taste

Nut Ricotta
100 g macadamia or cashew
2 tbsp nutritional yeast (optional)
2-3 tbsp plant based milk
2-3 tbsp lemon juice
1 tsp salt

Marinara
1 red onion
1 tbsp olive oil
4 pieces sun-dried tomatoes
100 g shredded tomatoes
1 tsp dried oregano
1/2 tsp chili flakes

Pesto
70 g fresh basil
50 g unroasted walnuts
1 tbsp olive oil
1 tsp pink himalayan salt
A pinch of cayenne

For the base, using a vegetable peeler or a mandolin, peel the zucchini thinly. Cut your tomatoes thinly. Cut flat bread in to squares. Set aside.

To make pesto sauce, place all pesto layer ingredients in a food processor, mix on high until until get a fluffy consistency.

For the marinara, place all tomato layer ingredients in a food processor, mix on high until smooth.

To make nut ricotta, place all nut ricotta layer ingredients in a food processor, mix on high until completely smooth. (If you don't consume nutritional yeast, remove it from the list. It will still work and you will get delicious tangy flavour with the lemon juice.)

To assemble, place a flat bread piece in the plate, add two zucchini slices on top. Start with macadamia cheese layer in order to prevent tilting over. Because its consistency is more intense than other layer sauces. When nut ricotta layer is done, add one more zucchini layer and sliced tomato then flat bread. Pour pesto sauce and add one more zucchini layer. Repeat and top with a final dollop of pesto and cheese. Decorate with oregano, or hemp hearts and edible flowers, if desired. Keep the lasagna in the fridge. It is best when consumed immediately.

ICARO'S PLATE

Yield: 3-4

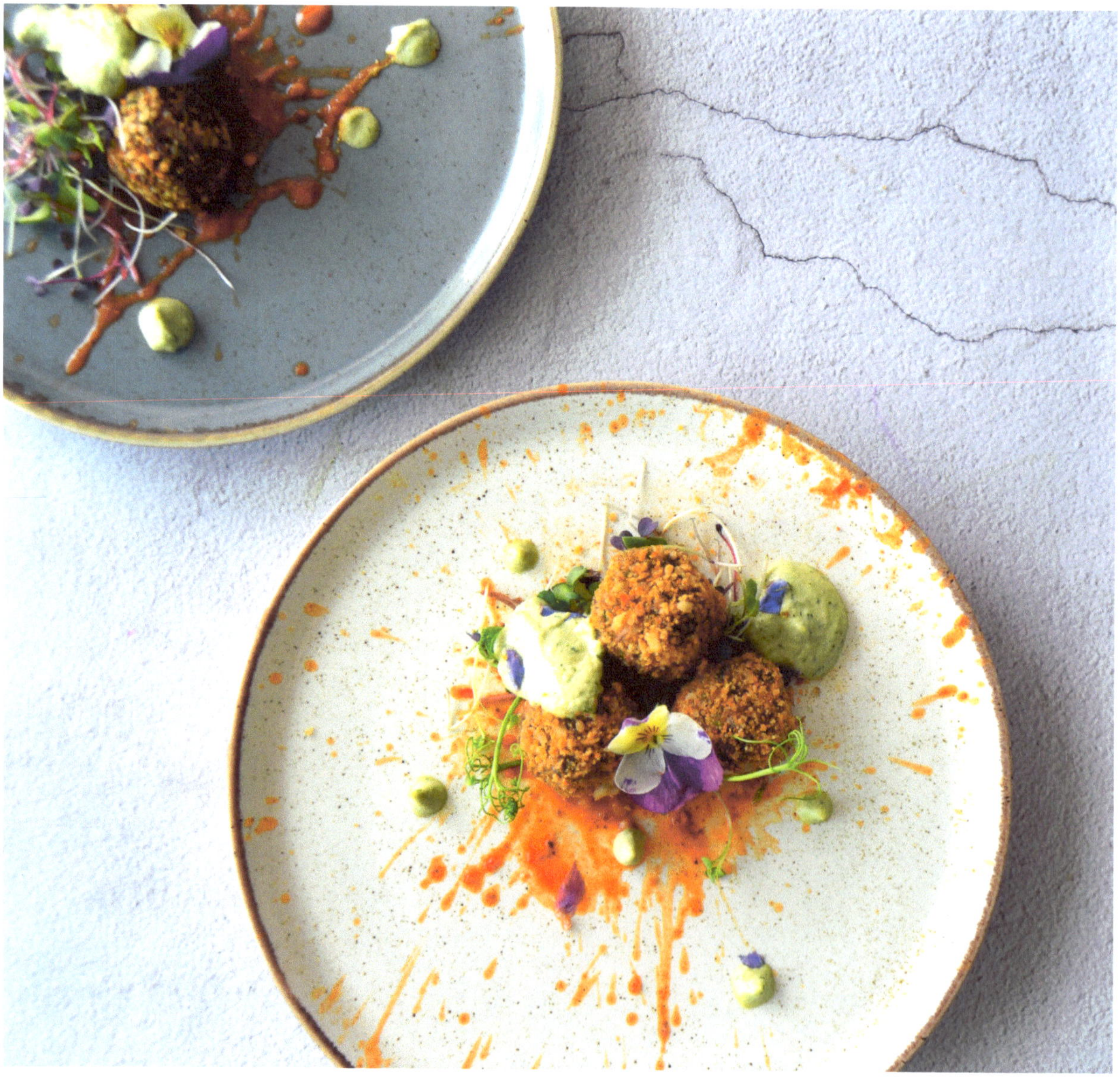

Pea Hemp Balls

55 g hemp hearts

175 g pea

2 tbsp dulse wakame nori mix

1 tbsp coconut aminos

1 tbsp olive oil

2 tbsp lemon juice

3 tbsp chia seeds + 9 tbsp water

1 tsp onion powder

1 tsp red pepper

1 tbsp agave or maple syrup

3 tbsp sprouted green lentil flour

Crumble

40 g soaked walnuts

1/4 tsp red pepper

2 tsp sweet paprika

Tartar Sauce

100 g cashews soaked

85 ml. water

A pinch flaked salt

A pinch black pepper

1 tbsp finely chopped parsley

1 tsp onion powder

2 tbsp pickled capers

1/4 cup finely chopped dill

1 tbsp apple cider vinegar

Sweet Chili

1 large red bell pepper chopped

1 jalapeno chopped

1 large tomato chopped

1/2 tsp salt

To make pea hemp hearts, place all pea hemp ball ingredients in the food processor, mix on high speed until combined well. Form dough into balls using a tablespoon or icecream scooper.

Grind crumble ingrediets in a food processor and transfer to a bowl. Coat balls in the crumbs and dehydrate for 6 to 8 hours at 42°C until completely dried.

To make chili, blend all ingredients well until silky smooth. Chill until ready to use. It will keep for up to 3 days in a sealed container in the fridge.

To make tartar sauce, Blend cashews, water and vinegar until smooth. Stir in remaining ingredients. Chill to firm up for about 2 hours.

Place all the chili ingredients in a blender. Blend until smooth. Set aside.

Place a tablespoon chili sauce in the middle of the plate, using the back of a tablespoon splash it around the plate if you want to decorate this way.

Place your pea hemp balls over the sauce. Pour tartar sauce using a teaspoon over the balls, and drop small dots around the balls. Decorate with edible flowers and microgreens. The pea hemp balls are best when freshly dehydrated and consumed in the same day. If you will use later, reheat in the dehydrator before serving.

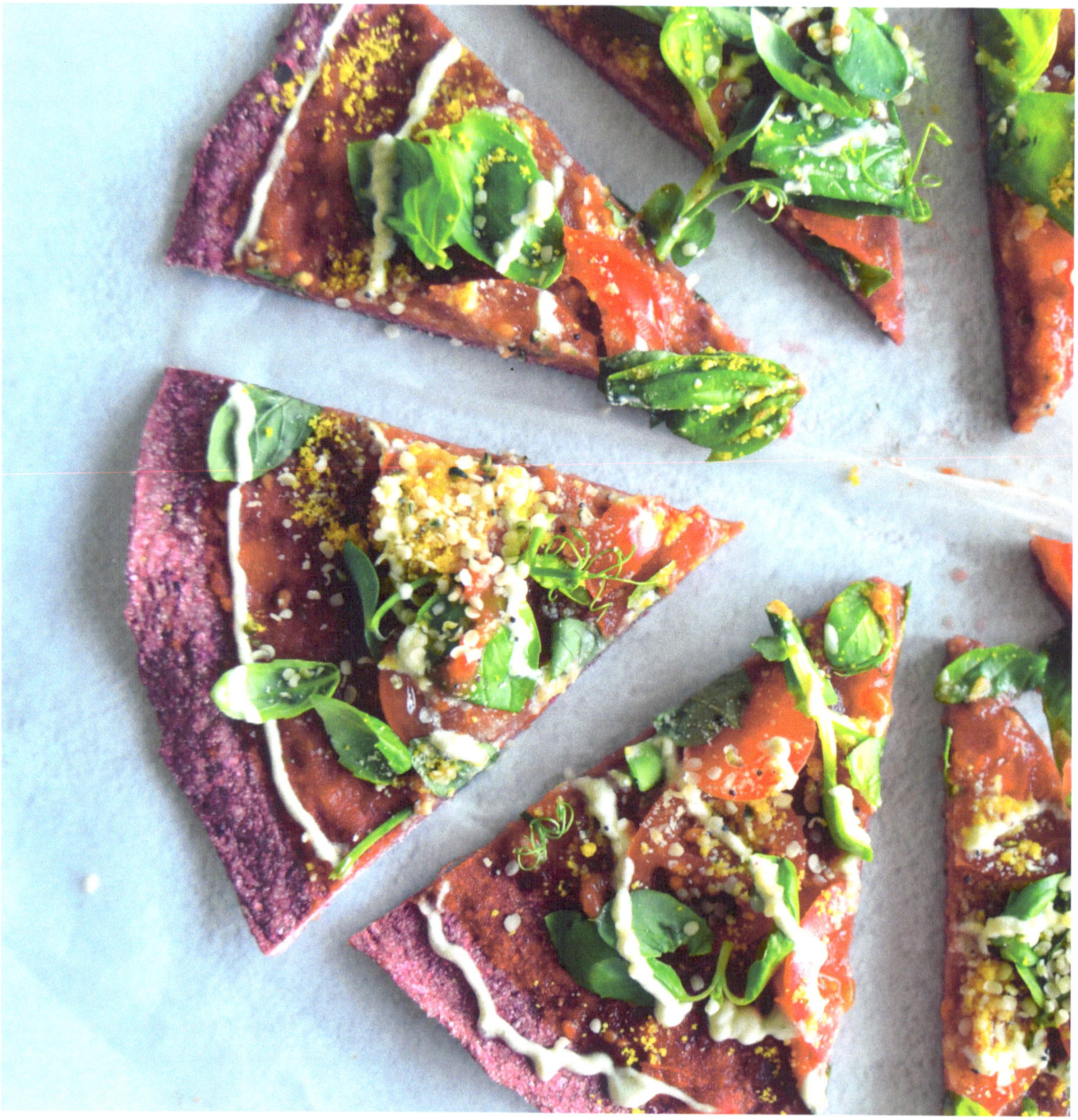

UNICORN PIZZA

Yield: 2 person

Crust
70 g sprouted buckwheat flour
20 g psyllium husk powder
1 tsp garlic powder
120 g beet puree
1/4 tsp salt
1/2 cup filtered water

BBQ Sauce
250 g tomato
2 medjool dates soaked in water
1 lemon juice
1 tsp paprika
1/4 tsp chili powder
1/2 tsp onion powder
1/2 tsp chipotle or red pepper flakes
1tsp garlic powder

Ranch Sauce
100 g raw cashew pre-soaked
1 tsp apple cider vinegar
2 tbsp chopped rosemary
1 tsp garlic powder
1/8 tsp black pepper
1/2 tsp himalayan salt
1/2 tsp onion powder
1/2 lemon juice
150 g filtered water

To make crust, wash the beets and slice into small cubes. Add to a high powered blender, mix on high speed until you get puree. Add the buckwheat flour, psyllium husk, garlic and water to the blender and blend until smooth. Make a ball, put mixture in the center of a paraflexx sheet lined dehydrator tray. Using a rolling pin, roll and give it a thin round shape. Dehydrate in the dehydrator at 42°C for 6-7 hours. Once the top is fully dry, flip the crust over on the tray and peel off the paraflexx sheet. Place the crust back into the dehydrator for 1-2 hours more until fully dry to the touch on both sides but not crispy.

To make BBQ, place all BBQ sauce ingredients into the food processor, mix well until smooth. Set aside.

To make ranch sauce, Place all ranch sauce ingredients into the blender, mix on high speed until you get silky smooth sauce. Pour in a bottle. Set aside.

To assemble, pour half of the BBQ sauce on top of the dried pizza crust. Spread evenly edge to edge . Slice the pizza into 6-7 pieces and carefully move the pizza slices back to the dehydrator tray. Keep the slices separated slightly.

Dehydrate at 40 C for 1-2 hours, turning the tray halfway through. Top with fresh basil tomato, rawmesan or whatever you want. Drizzle the with ranch sauce using a squeeze bottle on top and serve.

SPRING PIZZA

Yield: 3-4 person

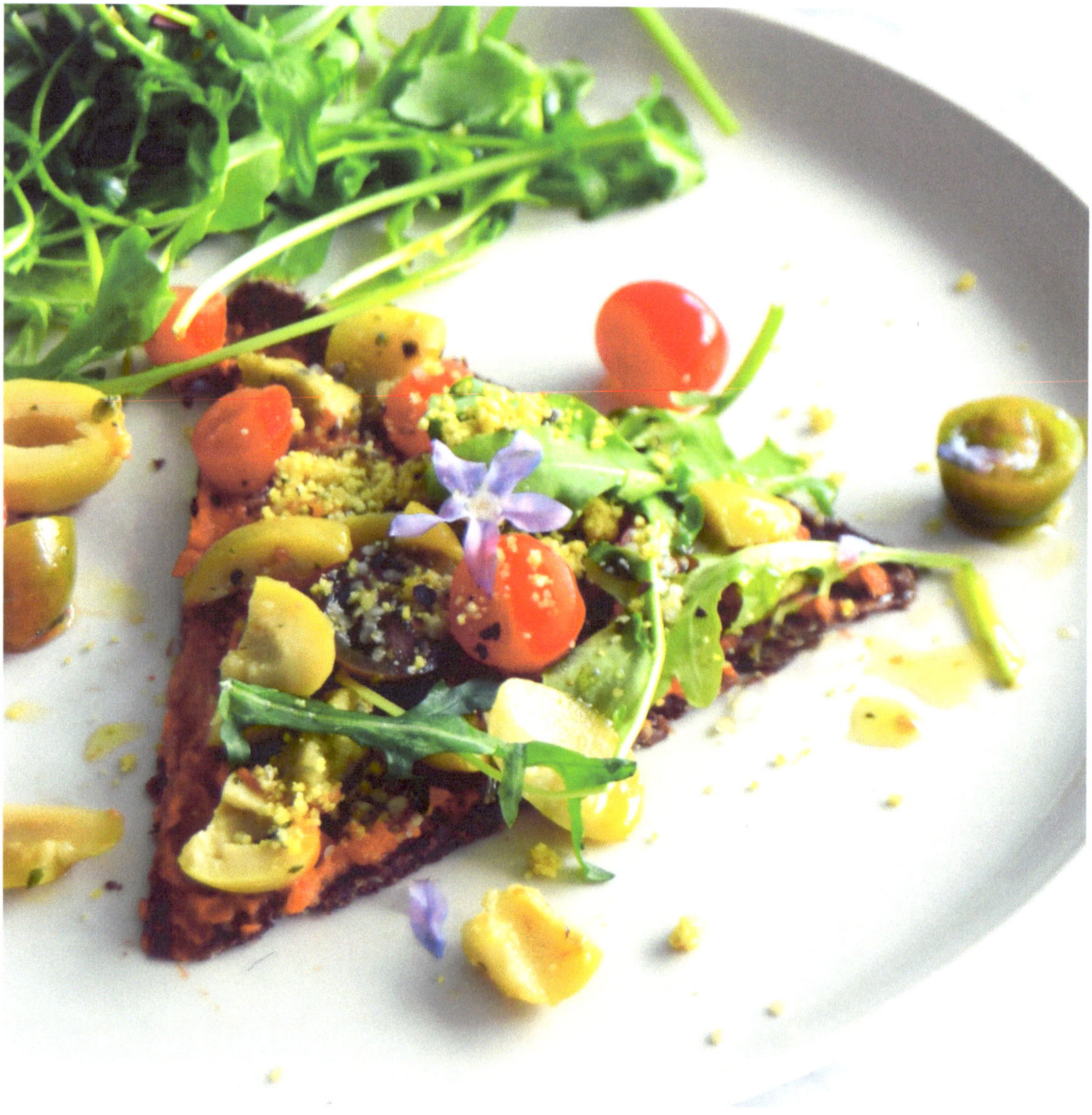

Base

3 cups walnut
1 cup ground flaxseed
1/2 cup water
1 tbsp olive oil
2 tbsp hemp hearts
1 tbsp dried basil
2 tbsp nutritional yeast (optional)
1 tbsp dried thyme
1/2 tsp himalayan salt
1 tsp onion powder
1 tsp garlic powder

Tomato Sauce

250 g tomato
7-8 sundried tomatoes
7-8 fresh basil leaves
A pinch of salt
1 tbsp olive oil

Toppings

Aged basil nut cheese
Fresh arugula
Rawmesan
Green olives
Cherry tomatoes
Borage flower to decorate

Place walnuts in food processor. Blitz until you get walnut meal. Basically, it should look almost as fine as flour. You are creating flour out of walnuts. Transfer flour in a bowl. Place flaxseed meal in a small bowl, add a little water , set aside for 10 minutes.

Add the rest of the ingredients and flax mixture to the bowl that contains the walnut meal. Stir and combine with a wooden spoon. Your recipe should now resemble the textu-re of pizza dough.
Make small pizza crusts. You want them quite thin, about 1/4 inch thick. Place your crusts on parchment paper inside your dehydrator.
Dehydrate at 42°C for 1 2 hours, then reduce heat to 30 C and dehydrate for another 7-10 hours or so. Halfway through dehydrating your raw pie crusts you should remove the parchment and flip the pie crusts over so that the air can circulate better. Dehydrate them until completely dry.

Place all tomato sauce ingredients into the food processor, mix well until smooth.

Cut your cheese into small pieces, wash and drain arugula, cherry tomatoes and olives. Set aside.

When your crust is completely dried, pour tomato sauce over the crust. Dehydrate additional 20-30 minutes. Then top with olives, cherry tomatoes, arugula and aged basil nut cheese.. Sprinkle rawmesan for extra taste and decorate with borage flowers if desired. Cut and serve!

CAULIFLOWER PIZZA

Yield: 3-4 person

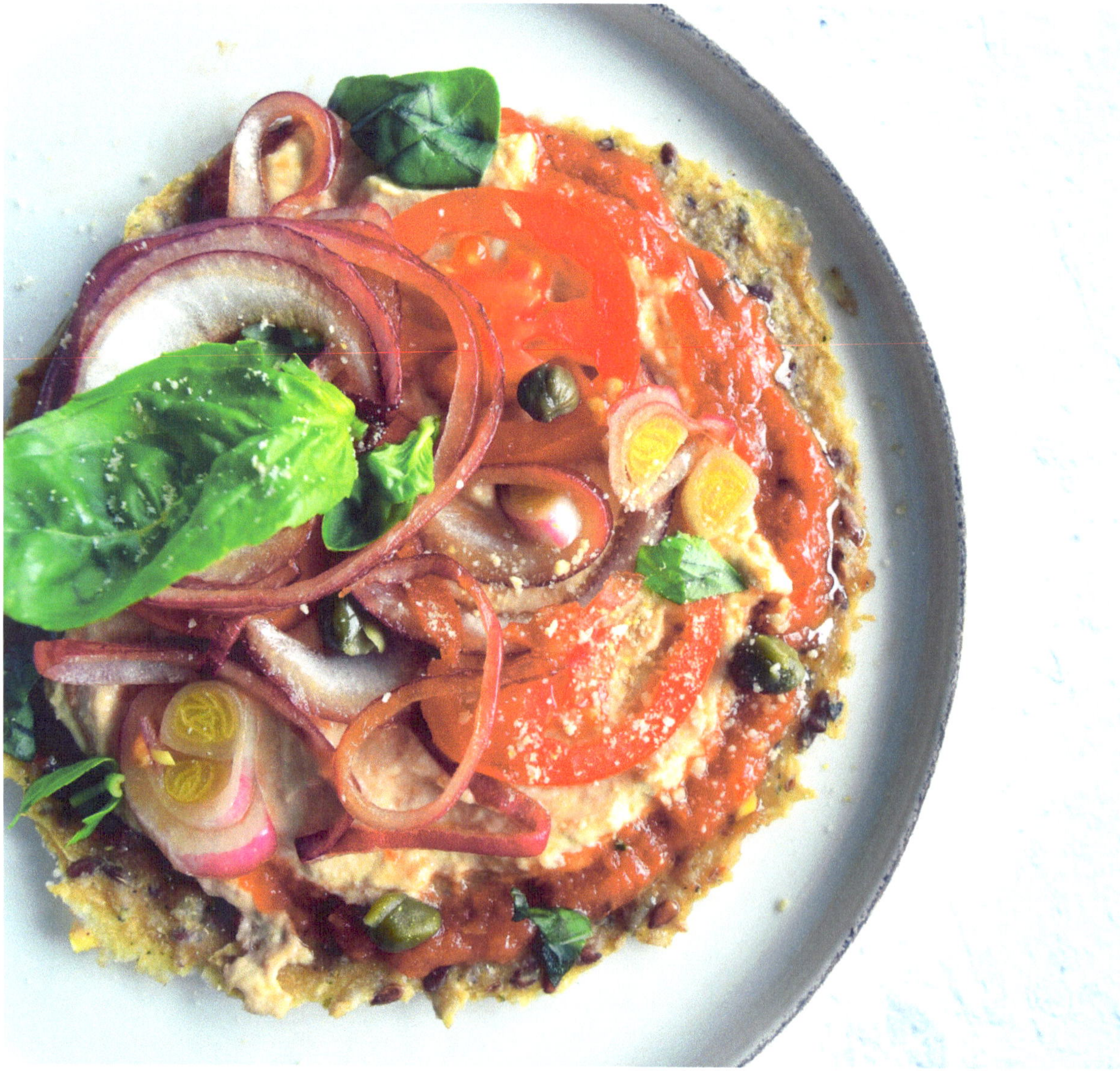

Base

310 g cauliflower broken into florets

50 g sunflower seeds

3 garlic cloves minced

2 tbsp flaxseed seeds

2 tbsp water

5-6 tbsp sprouted oat flour

1 tbsp psyllium seeds

3 tbsp hemp hearts

1 tbsp lemon juice

1/2 tsp sea salt

1 tbsp olive oil

2 tbsp nutritional yeast

1 tsp oregano

1/2 tsp red pepper

Sunflower Seed Cheese Cream

1 cup sunflower seeds

3 tbsp nutritional yeast

1 tsp garlic powder

1 tbsp coconut aminos

2 tbsp lemon juice

1/4 tsp salt

Tomato Sauce

1 cup cherry tomatoes

1/2 cup sundried tomatoes

1 tsp raw agave or syrup

1/4 tsp salt

Toppings

1 red onion thinly sliced

1 tbsp balsamic vinegar

1 tsp raw agave syrup

Cherry tomates sliced

1-2 tbsp capers

Fresh basil leaves

Place the cauliflower florets in a food processor, mix on high speed until you get rice-like texture.
Add the rest of ingredients, pulse to combine.
On a non-stick dehydrator sheet, pour 2 tbsp mixture into circles that are 1/4-inch thick or depending on how thin you like.

Dehydrate at 42°C for 4-6 hours. (I love my pizza crust very thin and it takes only 4 hours. If you spread thick, you will need to dehydrate longer.)

To make tomato sauce, place all ingredients into blender. Blend well until smooth. After 5-6 hours, pour mixture over the crust circles. Spread well, dehydrated for 20 minutes.

To make cheese spread place all ingredients in food processor and blend until smooth. Spread over the tomato sauce.

Toss sliced onions and tomatoes with balsamic vinegar and agave syrup.

Place onions and tomatoes on dehydrator sheets. Dehydrate for a hour. I do this while the crust is dehydrating. You want these wilted but not super dry.

Top with basil leaves, capers dehydrated tomatoes and onions. Serve immediately.

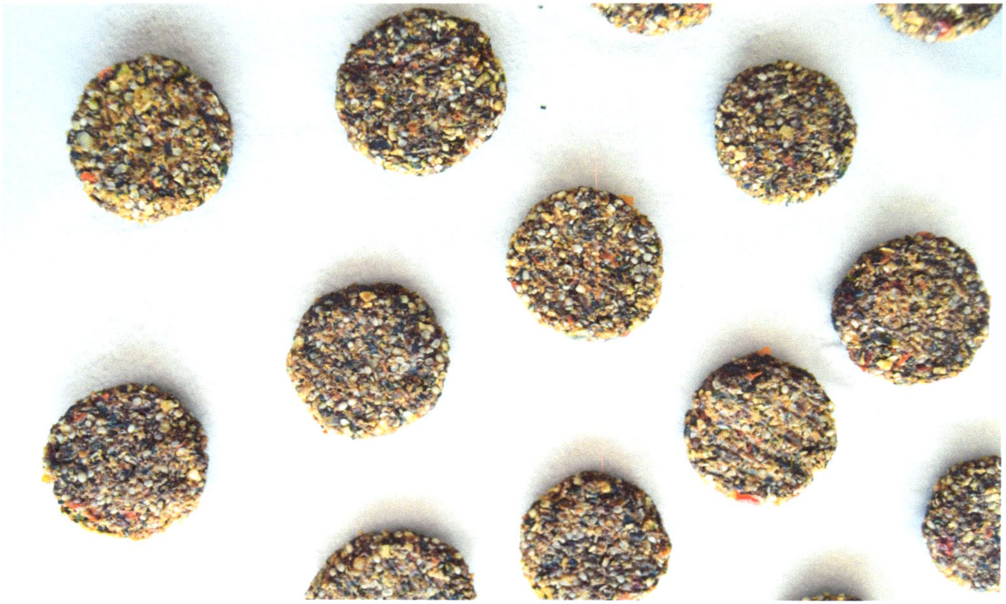

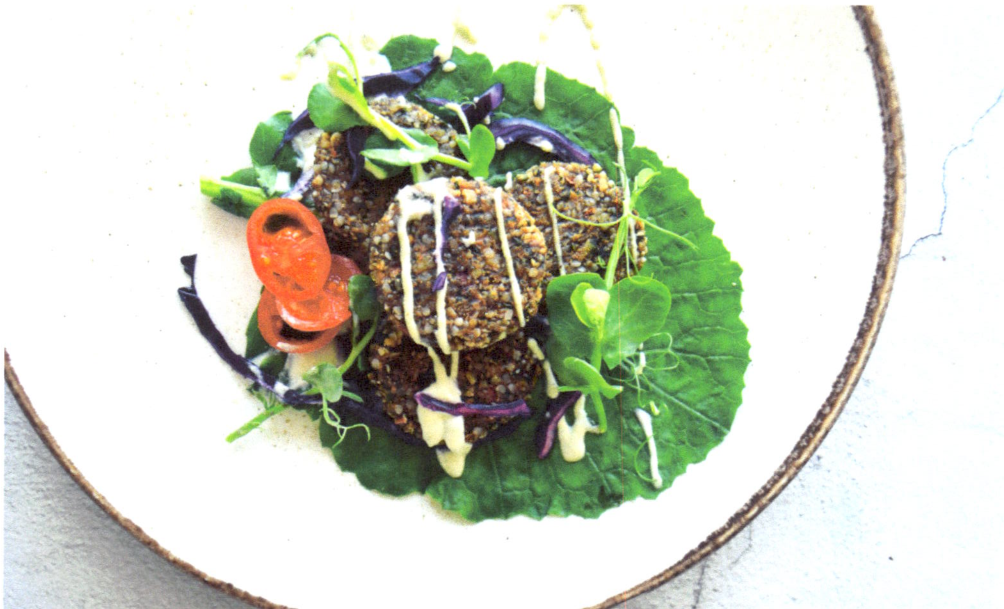

HEMP BURGER

Yield: 4-5 person

For the Hemp Burger

80 g hemp hearts
20 g ground flax seed
40 g sprouted mung bean flour
15 g chia seeds
65 g white onion
30 g green pepper
70 g red bell pepper
110 g tomatoes
A handful of fresh parsley
1 tsp garlic puree
1 tsp pink himalayan salt
75 g walnut crushed
70 g pumpkin seeds

For the Wrap

6-7 collard greens
4-5 cherry tomatoes
1/4 cup chopped purple cabbage
1/4 cup sprouted pea

For the Mint Cashew Dressing

100 g raw cashews pre-soaked
2 tbsp chopped fresh mint
1 tsp garlic powder
3 tbsp lemon juice
150 ml water
1/4 tsp onion powder
1/2 tsp pink himalayan salt

Start making cashew mint dressing first, place all ingredients into the food processor, mix on high speed until get silky smooth consistency. Pour mixture in a squeeze bottle or a glass jar.
Keep in the refrigerator at least 2 hours before using.
Store up to 5 days.

Wash and dry your collard greens, sprouted peas, tomatoes and purple cabbage. Cut your purple cabbage thinly. Set them aside.

Add all the hemp burger ingredients except hemp hearts to your food processor. Mix until well combined and transfer into a large bowl. Add hemp hearts and mix using a spoon.

Line your dehydrator trays with paraflexx sheets. Form patties into small balls with your hands, similar to burger patties - about 1/2 to 3/4 inch thick. Place on the trays.

Dehydrate at 46°C for 2 hours. Reduce heat to 30 degrees and dehydrate for another 2-3 hours or until dried and they reach desired consistency.

When burgers are done, place them into the collard greens, add sliced tomatoes, sprouted pea and purple cabbage. Spread cashew dressing over the patties. Roll and eat immediately. Can be stored in the refrigerator up to 3 days but best when consumed in the same day.

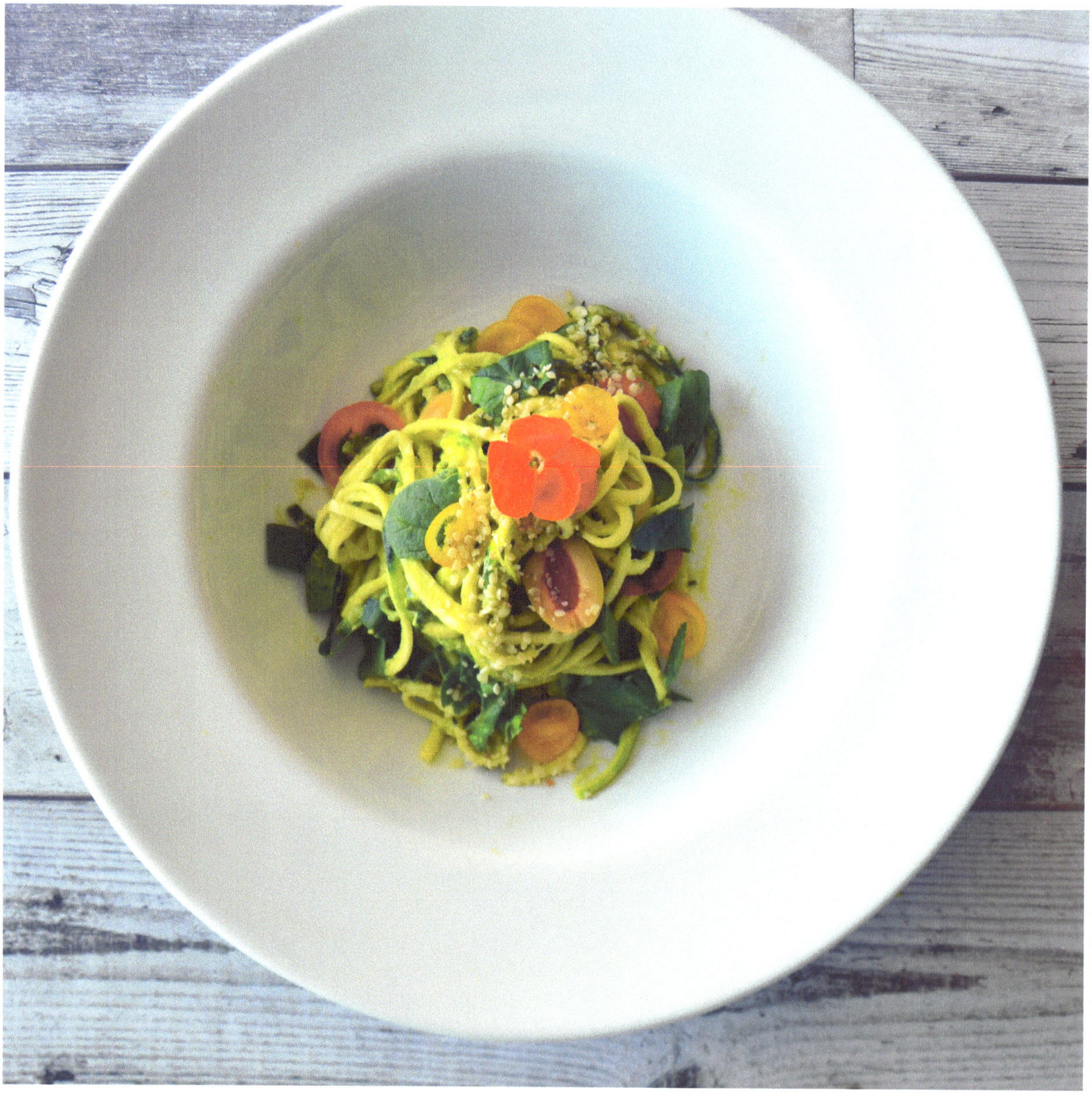

ZUCCHINI NOODLES

Yield: 3-4 person

Zoodle

3 large zucchini
1/2 cup green olives
1/2 cup cherry tomatoes
1 cup baby spinach

Sauce Ingredients

1 ripe large avocado
1 tsp garlic powder
5-6 fresh basil leaves
2 tbsp hemp hearts
4 tbsp almond milk
2 tbsp lemon juice
1 tsp salt

Sprilalize your zucchini. Set aside. Chop spinach leaves into small pieces.
Add in to a bowl with olive and halved cherry tomatoes together. Set aside.

Add peeled and cored avocado, garlic powder, almond milk, fresh basil, lemon juice and salt in to the food processor.

Mix on high speed until you get a smooth mixture. If you need add more almond milk or water to thin.

Pour dressing over salad and toss to coat.

Toss tomatoes, olives and spinach leaves with your zoodle. Sprinkle hemp seeds, decorate with edible flowers if desired and serve!

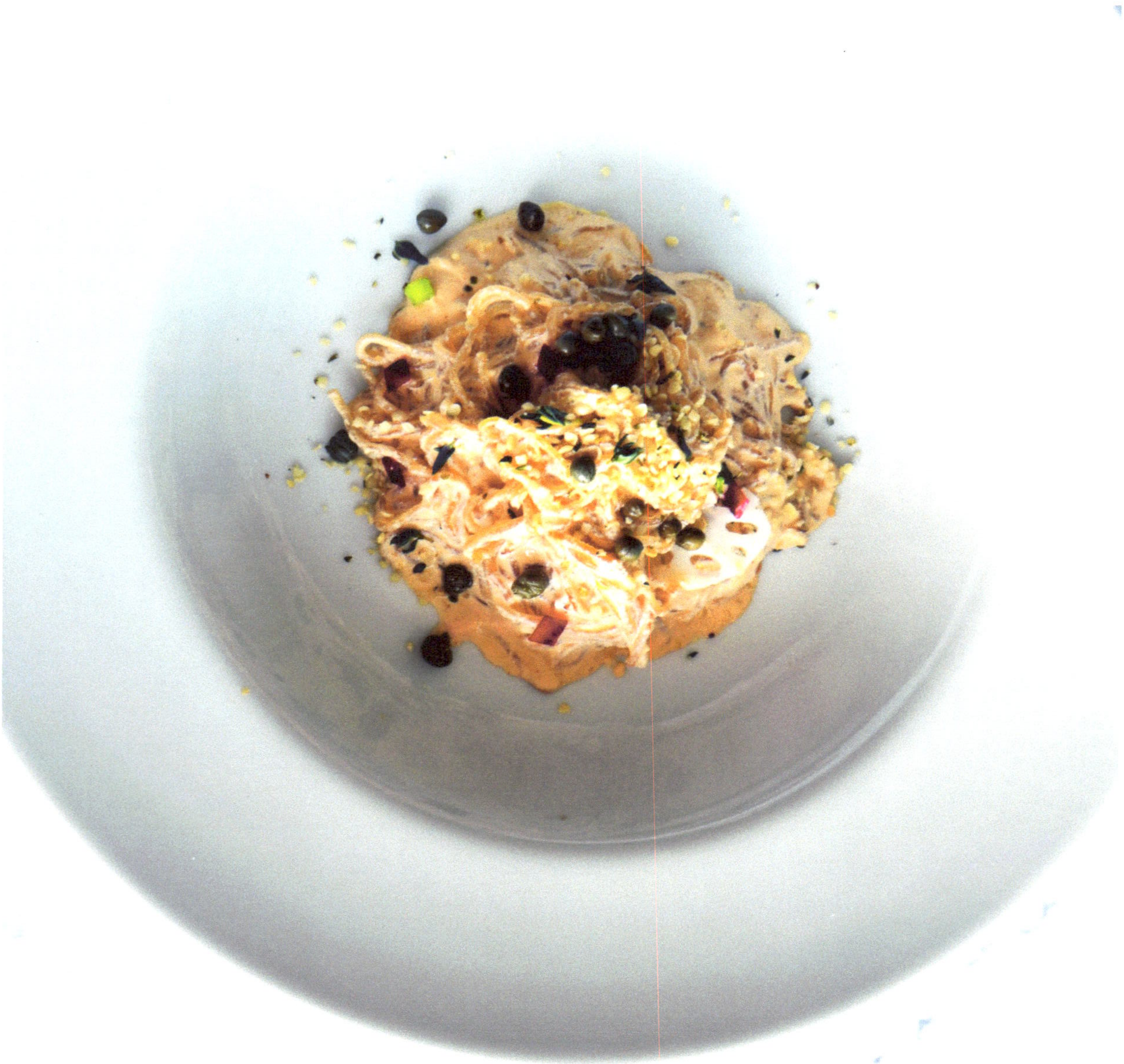

JUST MARRIED KELP NOODLE

Yield: 2 person

Marination

200 g kelp noodles
1 tsp baking soda
3 tbsp lemon juice
1 tbsp olive oil
1 tbsp coconut nectar
1 tbsp coconut aminos

Sauce

70 g raw cashews pre-soaked
50 ml filtered water
2 tbsp lemon juice
1 tsp pink himalayan salt
1 tsp chili pepper

Toppings

1 tbsp hemp hearts
1 tbsp capers

Thoroughly rinse kelp noodles and place into a large bowl. Add lukewarm water and baking soda and soak for 10 minutes. Drain and rinse well.
Add 1 tbsp lemon juice, olive oil, coconut nectar and coconut aminos, let it marinate for at least 1 hour.

To make sauce, In a high speed blender mix pre-soaked cashews with filtered water and 2 tbsp lemon juice. Then add sea salt, chili paper, stir well. (Use sunflower seeds or macadamia in the place of cashews if desired)

Toss your marinated kelp noodles with the sauce.
Divide between bowls. Sprinkle some hemp seeds and capers. Serve!

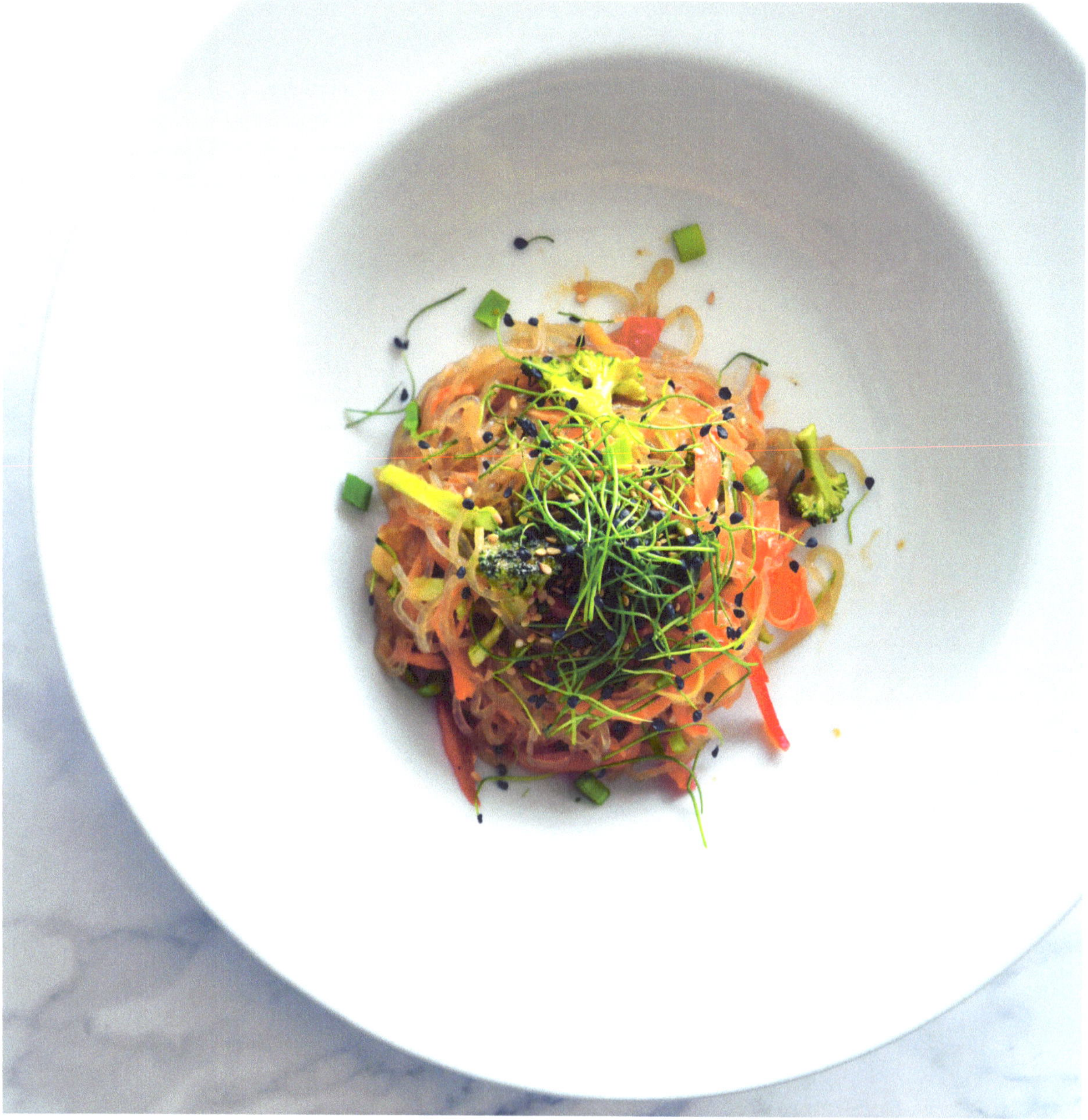

CARROT KELP NOODLE

Yield: 2-3 person

Noodle Base

250 g kelp noodles
2 medium carrots
1 cup broccoli florets
1 large red bell pepper

Sauce

3 tbsp coconut aminos
2 large medjool dates
1 tbsp sesame oil
1 tsp grated fresh ginger
3 tbsp orange juice
1 tsp pink himalayan salt

Toppings

1/2 cup chopped green onions
2 tsp sesame seeds
A handful of garlic microgreens or your favorite microgreens

In lukewarm water, rinse your noodles.
Dry and place in a large bowl. Cut carrots in spiralize shape using a spiralizer. Place in a medium bowl, add chopped broccoli, and thinly sliced red pepper. Toss gently, set aside.

Place all sauce ingredients in a high speed blender. Mix until completely smooth and the dates become paste.

Pour sauce over noodles and half over chopped vegetables. Cover and place in the refrigerator for about 2 hours to marinate. This process will make your noodles soft like cooked texture. Once marinated place vegetables and noodles into strainer, remove excess sauce to drain out.

Garnish with green onions, sesame and garlic microgreens. Serve!

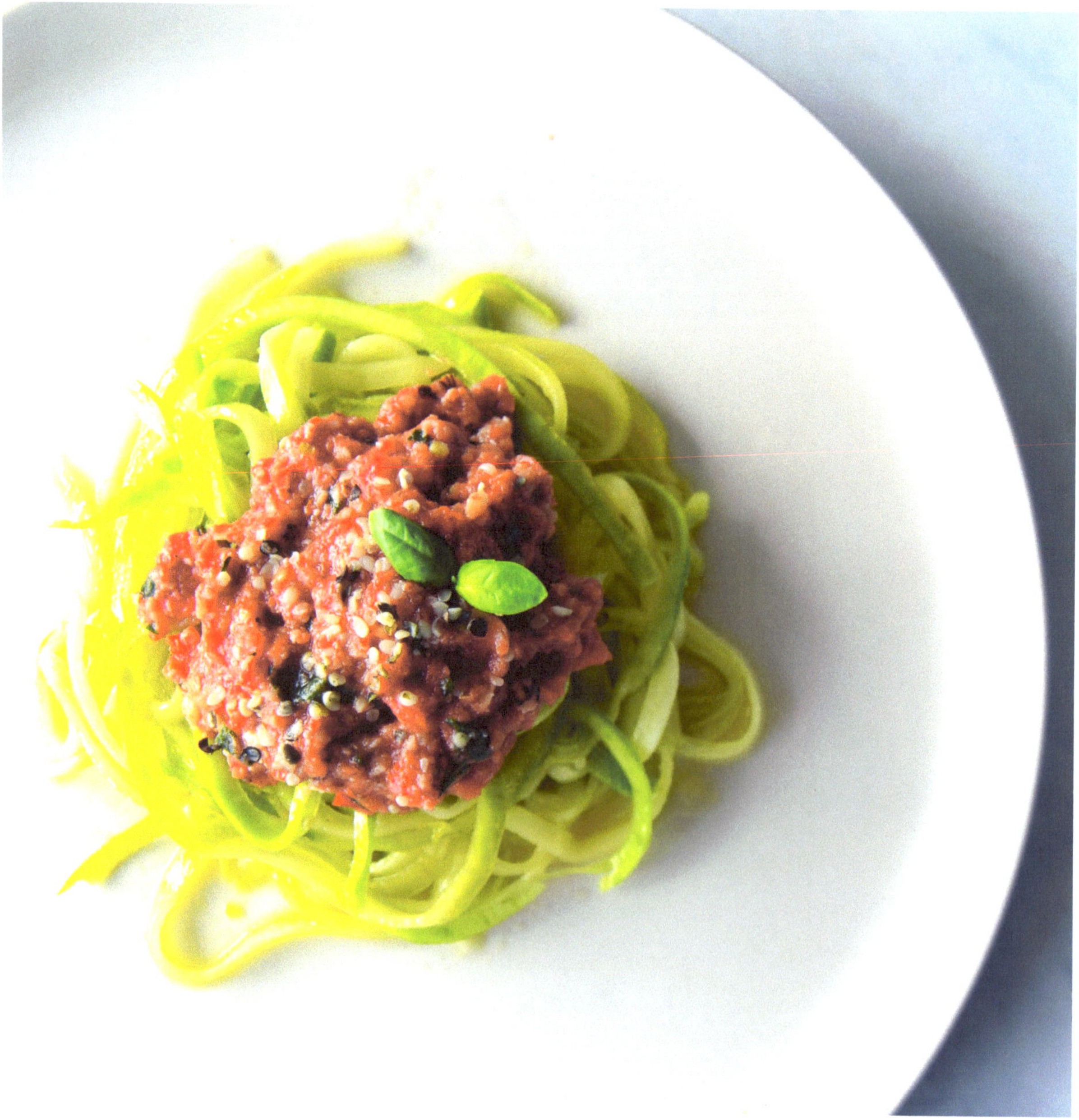

CLARITY OF BOLOGNESE

Yield: 3-4 person

Zoodle
4 large zucchini

Bolognese
300 g tomatoes
80 g walnuts
30 g sundried tomatoes
3-4 large fresh basil leaves
1/2 tbsp date or coconut nectarsyrup
1/4 tsp himalayan salt
Hemp hearts to serve

Using a spiral slicer, cut zucchinis into noodles.

Place walnuts into blender, process until chopped. You want them chopped not flour texture. Remove from the blender. Set aside. Add sundried tomatoes, basil leaves, and tomatoes, date syrup and salt into the blender. Mix until you get smooth texture. Then remove mixture and pour over the walnuts. Toss well.

Place zoodles in a bowl, Top with bolognese sauce, sprinkle hemp hearts and serve!

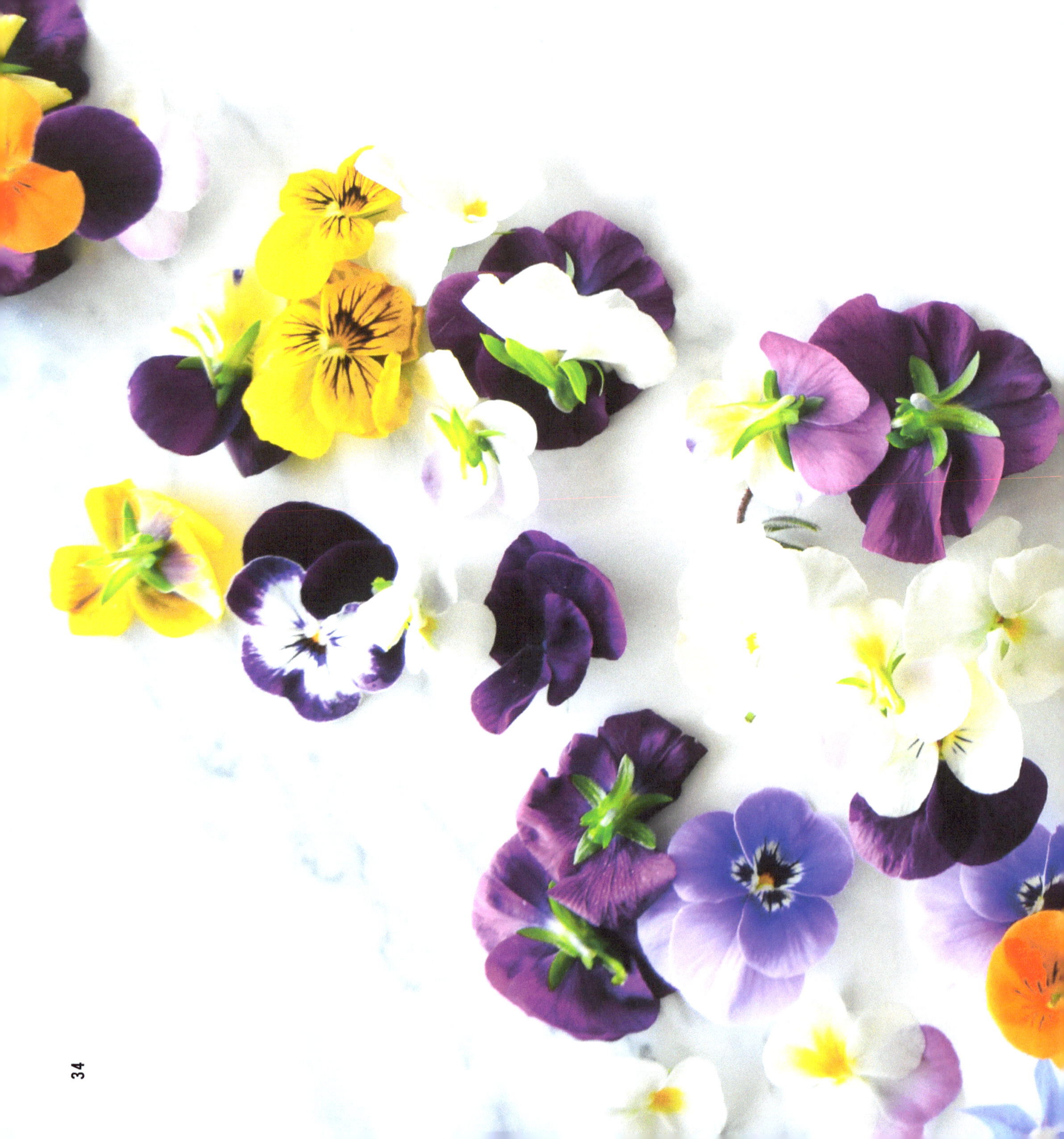

COMMON EDIBLE FLOWERS

WHAT THEY TASTE LIKE?

Scientific name: Tropaeolum
Flavor profile: Slight sweetness, pepper, spice, bitterness

Scientific name: Borago officinalis
Flavor profile: Mineral, cucumber, oyster

Scientific name: Viola tricolor hortensis
Flavor profile: Mild citrus, mint

Scientific name: Calendula
Flavor profile: Pepper

Scientific name: Eruca sativa
Flavor profile: Pepper, spice, grass

Scientific name: Lavandula
Flavor profile: Sweet, aromatic, herbaceous

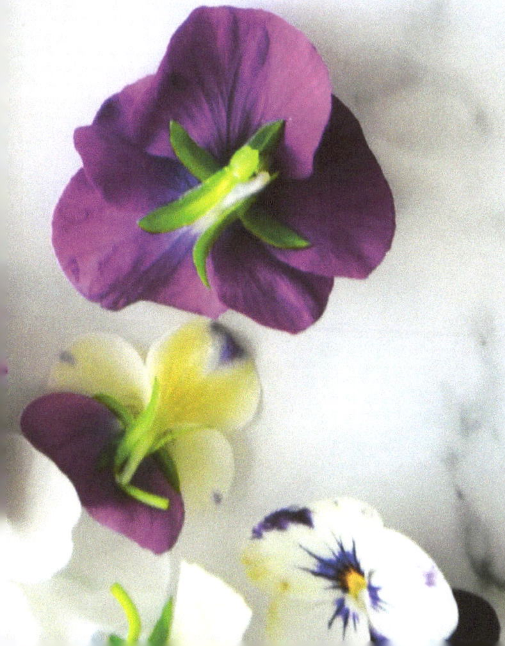

"RAW FOOD IS THE BEST WAY TO HAVE THE CLEANEST ENERGY!"

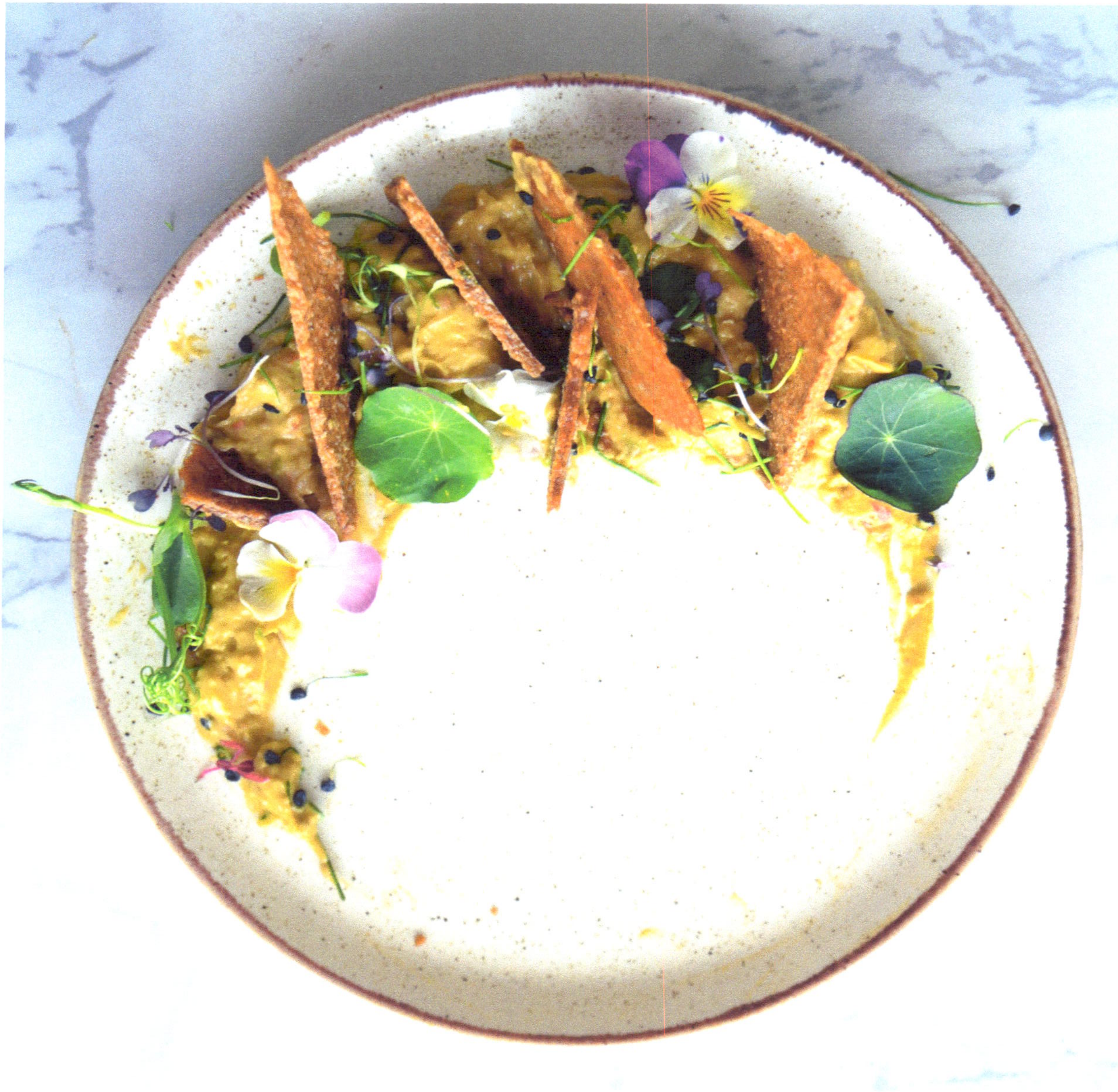

GOLDEN AGE OF RACHOS

Yield: 2-4 person

Rachos

110 g sunflower seeds
50 g sundried tomatoes
25 ml tomato juice or water
2 tbsp coconut aminos
1/4 tsp chili pepper
1/2 tsp ground coriander
1 tsp garlic powder
1 tsp onion powder
10 g spring onions
2 tbsp tbsp

Avocado Dip

1 ripe avocado
1/2 cup tomato juice
2 large sundried tomatoes
1/2 small chopped red onion
1 tbsp lemon juice
1 garlic clove minced
1/2 tsp pink himalayan salt

In a food processor, mix all rachos ingredients. Process on high until you get a smooth mixture.

Spread mixture directly onto a mesh dehydrator sheet leaving plenty of gaps between pieces of the mixture so the air can flow round nicely.
Give them a triangle shape using a knife or shape.

If you are using excalibur dehydrator use another dehydrator sheet to shape the crackers in triangle, after spreading the mixture over the dehydrator sheet, press down using another sheet then remove. This is super easy way to make them. Dehydrate for 12 hours or until completely dried.

To make avocado dip, mix all ingredients in a food processor until smooth.

Place your sauce in the plate drawing a lunate. Place the rachos triangles over the sauce. Decorate with sprouted garlic, nasturtium, edible flowers or whatever you want.

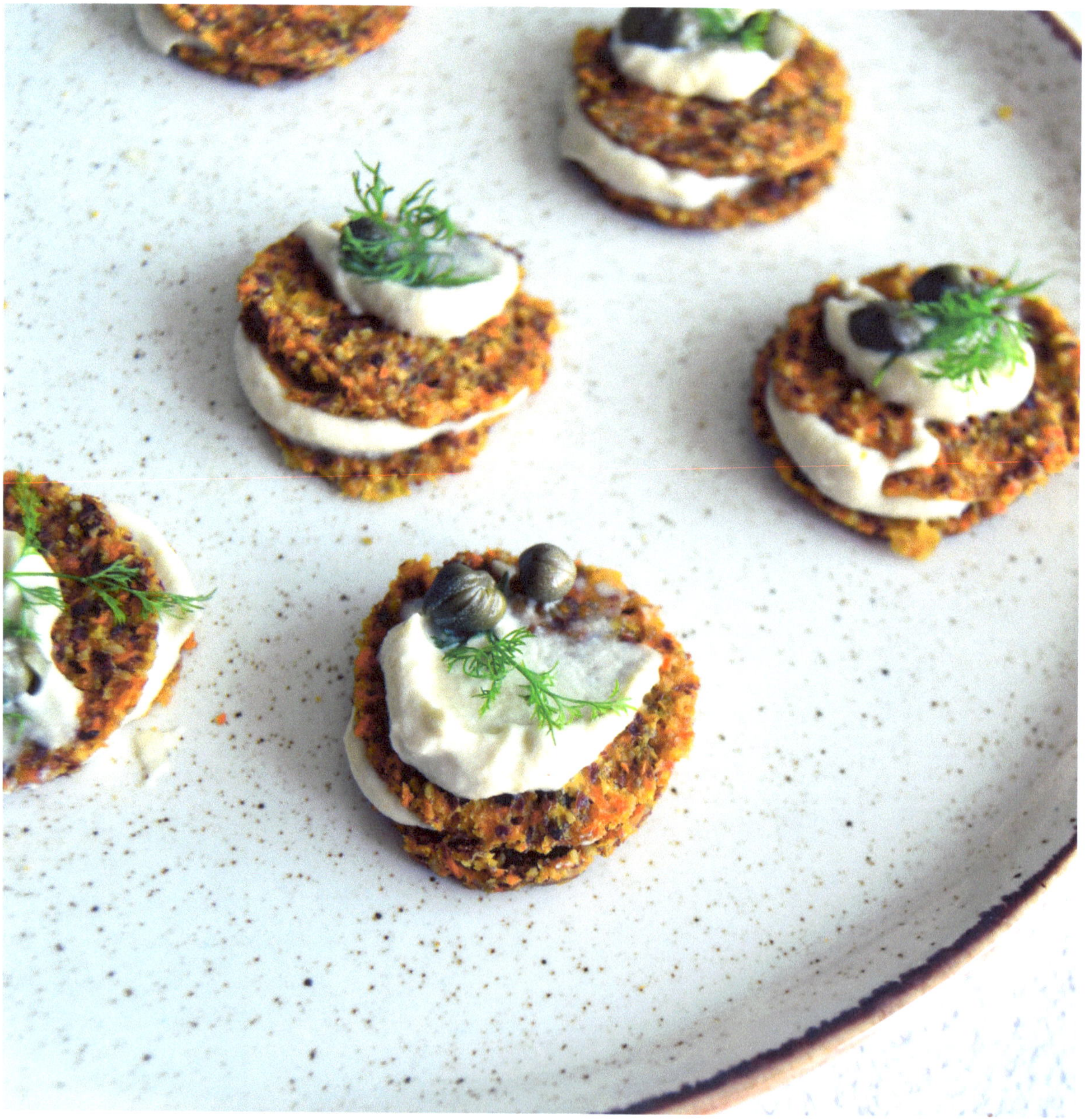

HARPA CANAPES

Yield: 4-6 person

Ingredients

1 cup carrots
1 medium red onion chopped
1 cup ground flaxseed
1 cup almond meal
1 cup water
2 tbsp nutritional yeast
1 tsp garlic powder
1/4 tsp chili powder
1 tsp pink himalayan salt
1 tbsp olive oil
1/4 cup capers and fresh dill to decorate

To make the carrot puree, simple blend the carrots and 1 cup water, then add the rest of the ingredients. Blend until you get sticky dough texture.

Spread evenly onto a dehydrator teflex sheet
Dehydrate at 42˚C for two hours, at this point, remove from the dehydrator, place another teflex sheet and tray over the top, carefully flip over and peel the original teflex sheet off so that you can dry the under side of the wrap.
Turn down the temperature to 35˚C and continue to dehydrate for a further three hours.

When your bread is dried completely, using a round cutter, cut them. Spread cashew cream cheese using a teaspoon. Put a lid and close canapes, spread cashew again. Put capers and fresh dill on top. Serve!

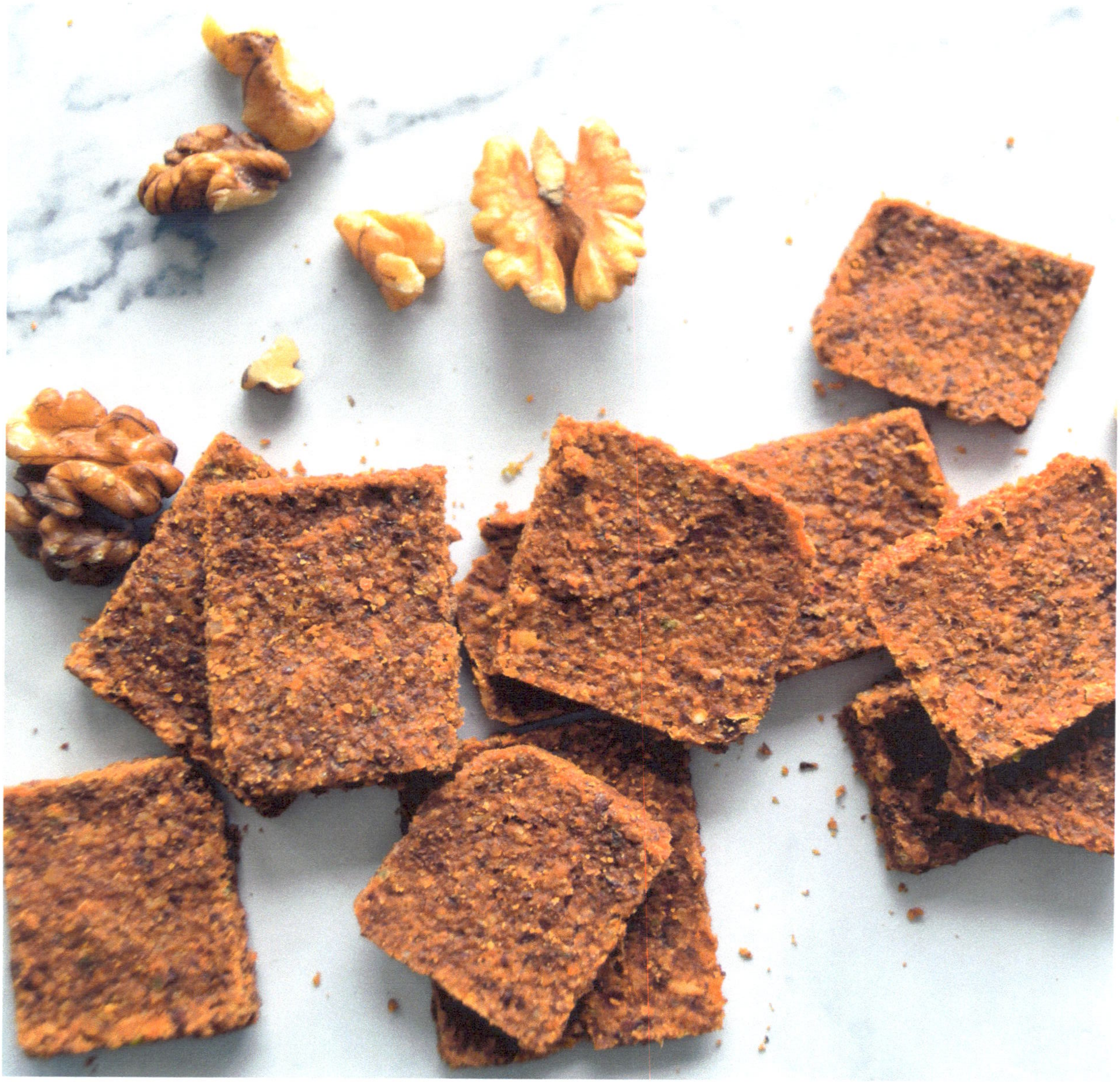

THE GATE CRACKERS

Yield: 2-4

Ingredients

90 g walnut soaked
40 g ground flaxseed
100 ml filtered water
1/3 cup sundried tomatoes
1/4 cup green olives
1 tsp dried oregano
1/2 tsp pink himalayan salt

Place the walnuts in the food processor and pulse until they are ground fine. Add the flax meal. Set aside.

Separately blend the sun-dried tomatoes, salt, oregano, water and olives, add to your walnut-flax flour mixture and mix by hand. Stir in the spices.

When it is done and become sticky dough, spread onto dehydrator sheet lined parchment paper. Press to 1/4th inch thick.

Dehydrate at 42°C for 1.5-2 hour, then turn to 35 C and dehydrate overnight until completely dried. You will want to flip the crackers half way through the dehydration process.

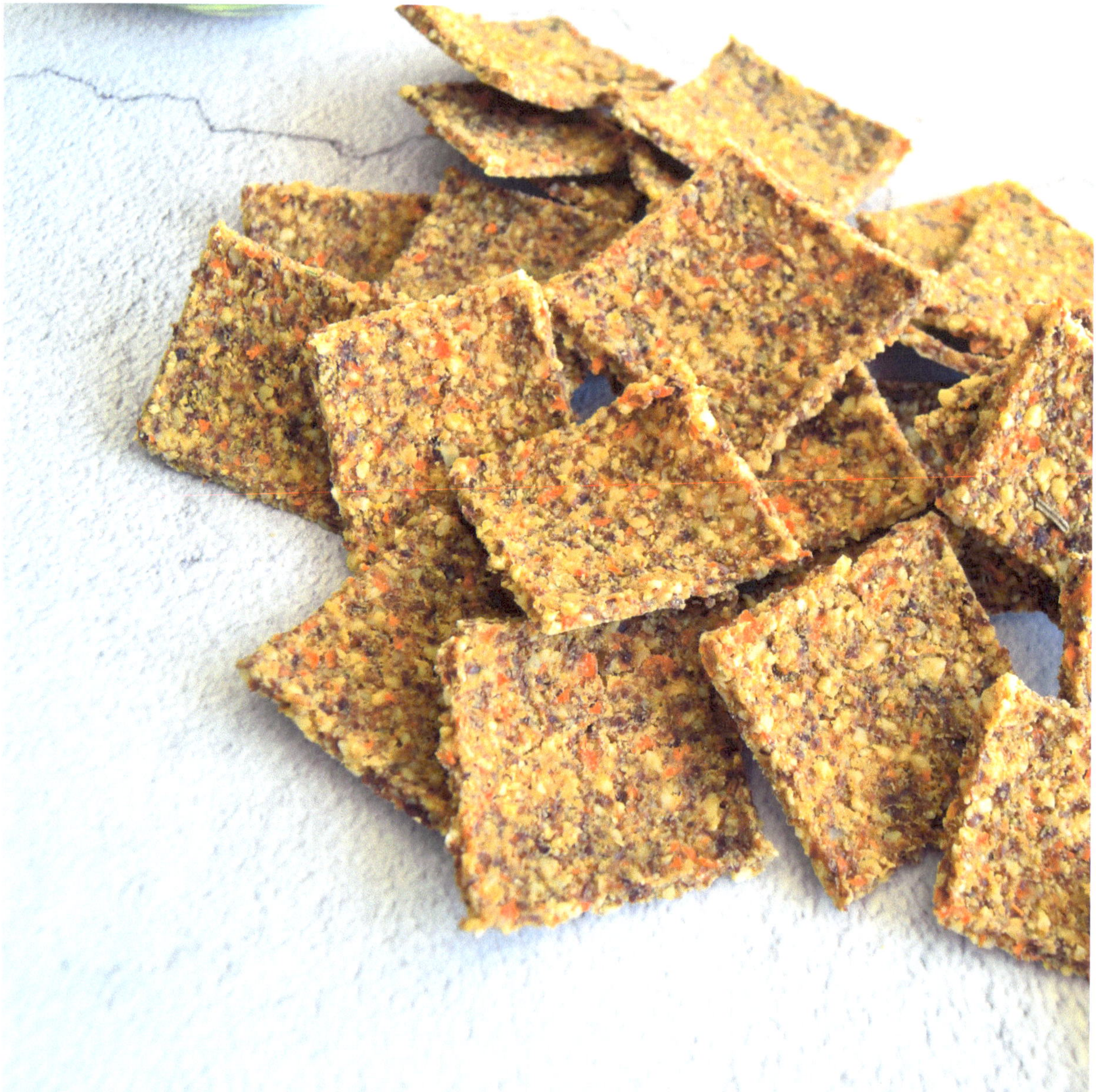

RISING CARROT CRACKERS

Yield: 4-6

Ingredients

1 cup ground flaxseed
1/4 cup coconut flour
4 tbsp nutritional yeast
2 medium carrots
1 cup cashews soaked
1/2 cup almonds
2 tbsp coconut oil
1 cup water
1 tbsp coconut nectar
2 tbsp coconut aminos
1 tsp pink himalayan salt

In a large bowl, combine the flaxseed meal, salt, coconut flour and the nutritional yeast. Set aside.

In a food processor, grind the almonds and cashews into a crumbly meal - don't over process. Transfer mixture into flaxseed bowl.

Process the carrots with coconut nectar until you have a nice mash. Scrape the mixture into the flaxseed bowl. Add the remaining ingredients and stir until thoroughly mixed. The mixture should be moist but hold together when pressed.

Divide the mixture in two and spread the half on a dehydrator tray that has been covered with a non-stick drying sheet. You'll just about be able to cover the full sheet. To get an even surface, I cover the dough with another non-stick sheet and gently roll with a rolling pin. Carefully lift off the non-stick sheet. Once the dough has been rolled out, gently score the surface into squares.

Place the trays in the middle of the dehydrator and set the temperature to 42°C. Dehydrate for 30 minutes, then reduce the heat to 35 C and dehydrate for an additional 6-8 hours or until the cracker are very crispy all the way through.

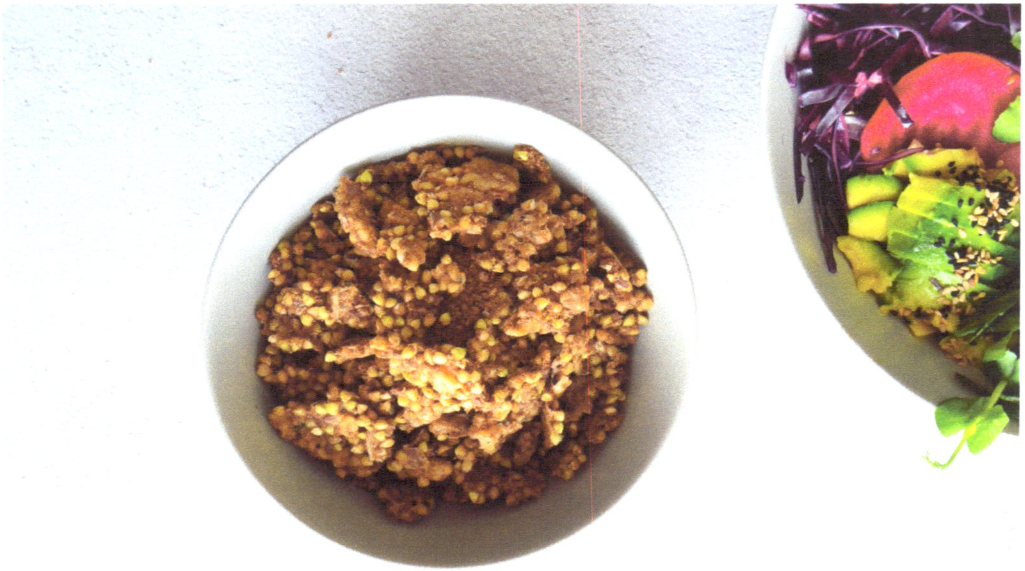

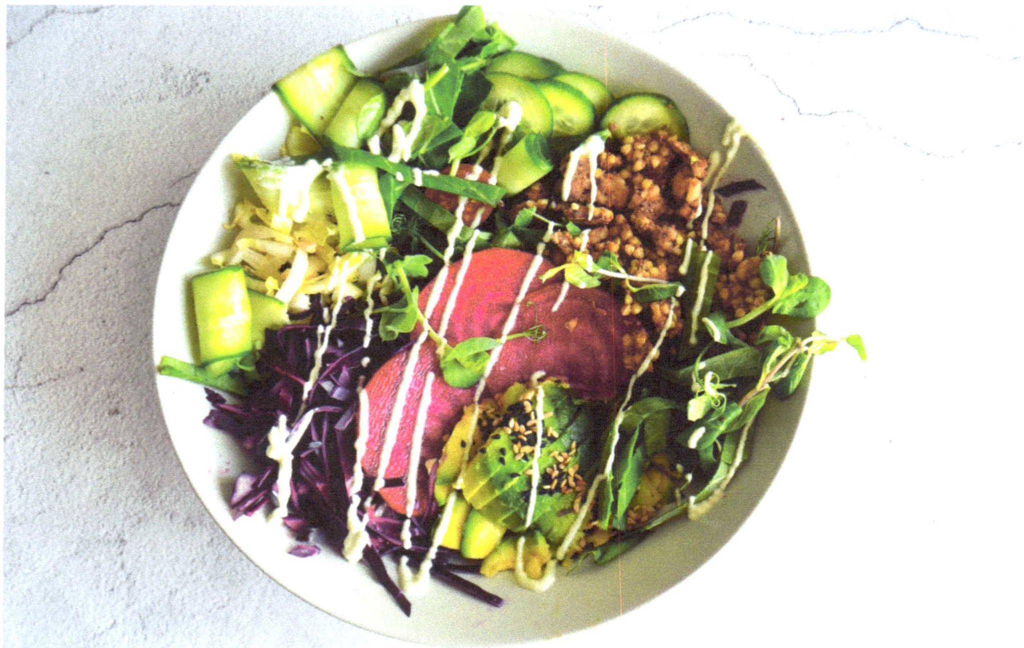

MUTUAL SAVORY RAWNOLA

Yield: 4-6 person

Rawnola

3 tbsp ground flaxseed
60 g raw walnuts
235 g raw buckwheat groats

Savory Paste

6 tbsp filtered water
1 tbsp olive oil
1 tsp paprika
1/2 tsp chili powder
1/2 tsp pink himalayan salt
1 tsp dried basil
1 tsp tomato
1 tsp garlic powder
1/2 tsp onion powder

Soak buckwheats in filtered water for 6 hours, then rinse and dry. Spread over the dehydrator tray lined parchment paper, then dehydrate at 42 degrees until completely dried.

In a small bowl, add 6 tbsp water and ground flax seed. Mix together set aside for 10 minutes.
Then transfer flax mixture in a large bowl. Add the olive oil, paprika, water, chili pepper, salt, basil, tomato powder, garlic and onion powder. Mix together.

Add the buckwheat and walnuts into the paste bowl. Toss together until combined well. Combine all ingredients together well.

Using a spatula, spread mixture onto the parchment paper. Dehydrate for 2 hours at 42°C then flip and dehydrate again for about 2-3 hours or until completely dried. Serve on the top of your salad and enjoy!

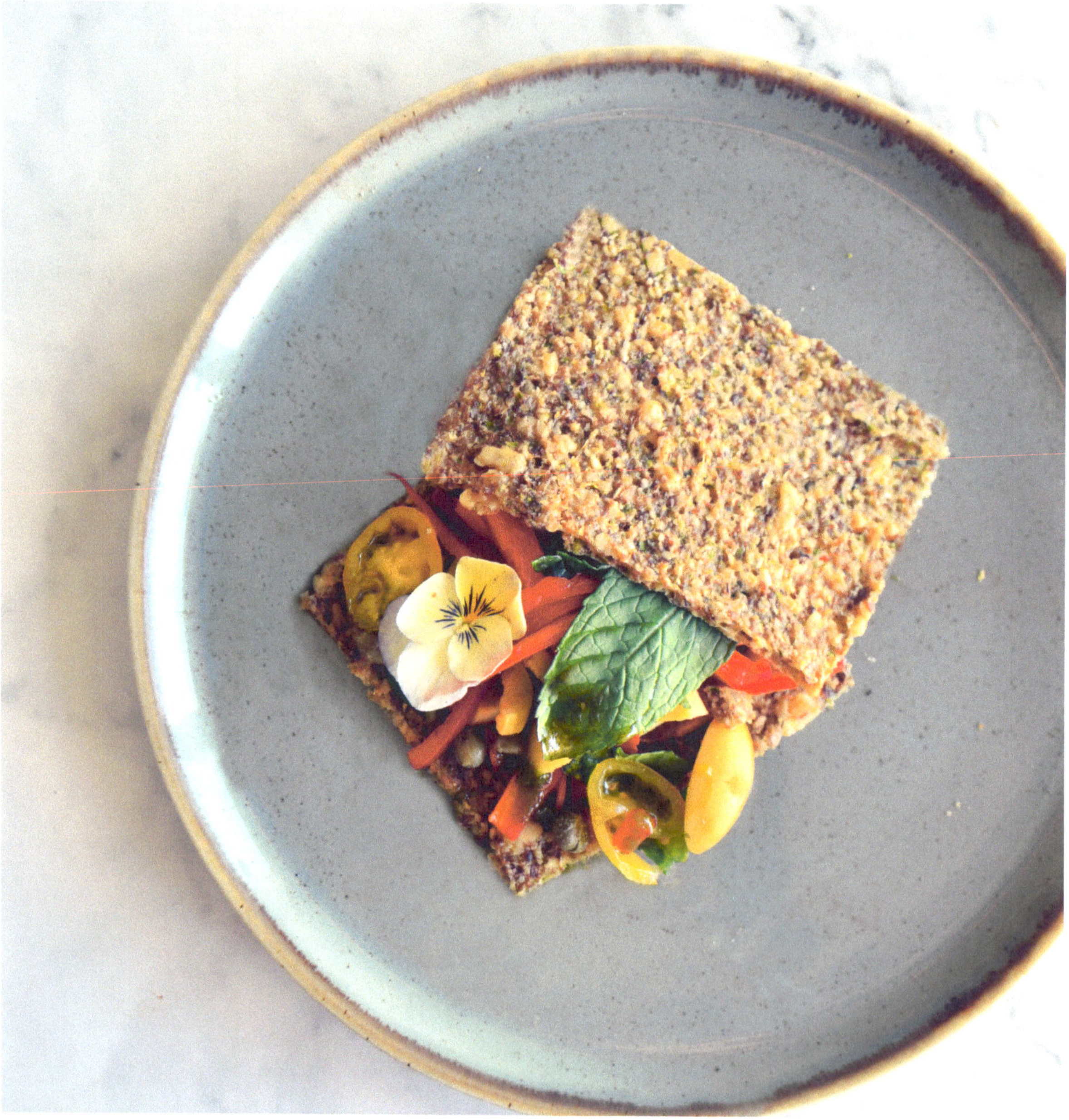

FROM CHAOS TO COSMOS TOAST

Yield: 2 person

Toast

1 small white onion
3 tbsp olive oil
1 medium zucchini
1 cup walnuts
2 medium dates pitted
4 tbsp ground flaxseed
1/2 tsp pink himalayan salt
1 tsp dried rosemary

Filling

2 tbsp kalamata olives
1 tbsp capers
1/2 cup red bell pepper
1/2 bunch fresh basil
1 cup tomatoes
2-3 slices aged raw nut cheese

Chop the onion and transfer to the food processor. Add the olive oil, zucchini, walnuts, dates, and salt. Blend until well combined, pulse a few times if there are a still chunks. Transfer to a bowl, stir in the ground flax seeds, and set aside to thicken, about five minutes.

Divide olives in two, cut red bell peppers julienne. Wash and dry your fresh basil leaves. Slice tomatoes very thin. Set aside.

Spread the mixture onto teflex sheets, about 1/4- to 1/2-inch thick, then cut into desired shapes and dehydrate for 12 to 24 hours. You may want to turn them after 8 hours. Put your crust on a nice serving platter or a cutting board, spread your favorite sauce or cheese on, and top with fillings. Eat immediately.

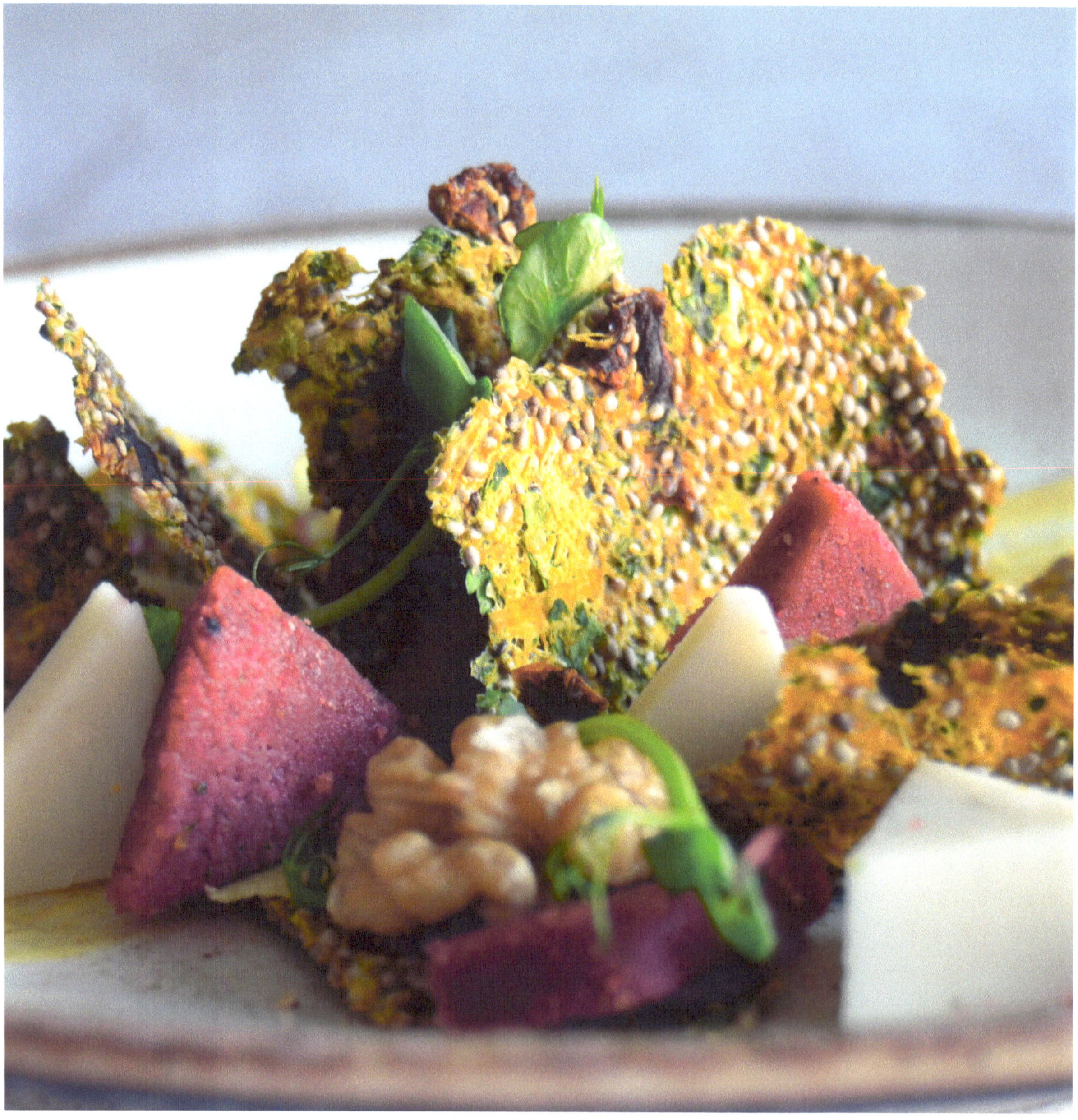

ZERO WASTE CELERY CRACKERS

Yield: 3-4 person

Ingredients

100 g flax seeds
1/2 cup celery pulp - leftovers from the celery juice
1/2 cup sundried tomatoes
80 g sunflower seeds
50 g chia seeds
1 teaspoon pickled capers
2 tbsp chopped green olives
75 g red onion chopped
55 g red pepper chopped
1 tbsp provence herbs
1 tsp garlic

Soak the flax seeds in a bowl and chia seeds in a seperate-bowl for 20 minutes.

Place the onion and red peppers, pulp leftovers from the celery juice, olives and sundried tomatoes into the food processor and mix until smooth.

Then add the capers, garlic, all herbs and soaked seeds. Thoroughly mix all ingredients together until the cracker mix is evenly combined. Scoop out your mixture onto dehydrator sheets and evenly spread the mixture.

Score your crackers into the shape and size you'd like them using a spatula, round cutter or triangle.

Set your dehydrator to 42 degrees and dehydrate for 8-10 hours. (If the crackers aren't dry enough flip them over and dry for an additional 6-8 hours.)

TIPS

If you haven't juiced, you can also just put celery in your food processor until it's completely broken down and pour it into your bowl with the other ingredients. If you do this rather than using veggie pulp, the crackers may take longer to dehydrate because the mixture will contain more water. You want the crackers very thin, so no more then 1/8 of an inch.

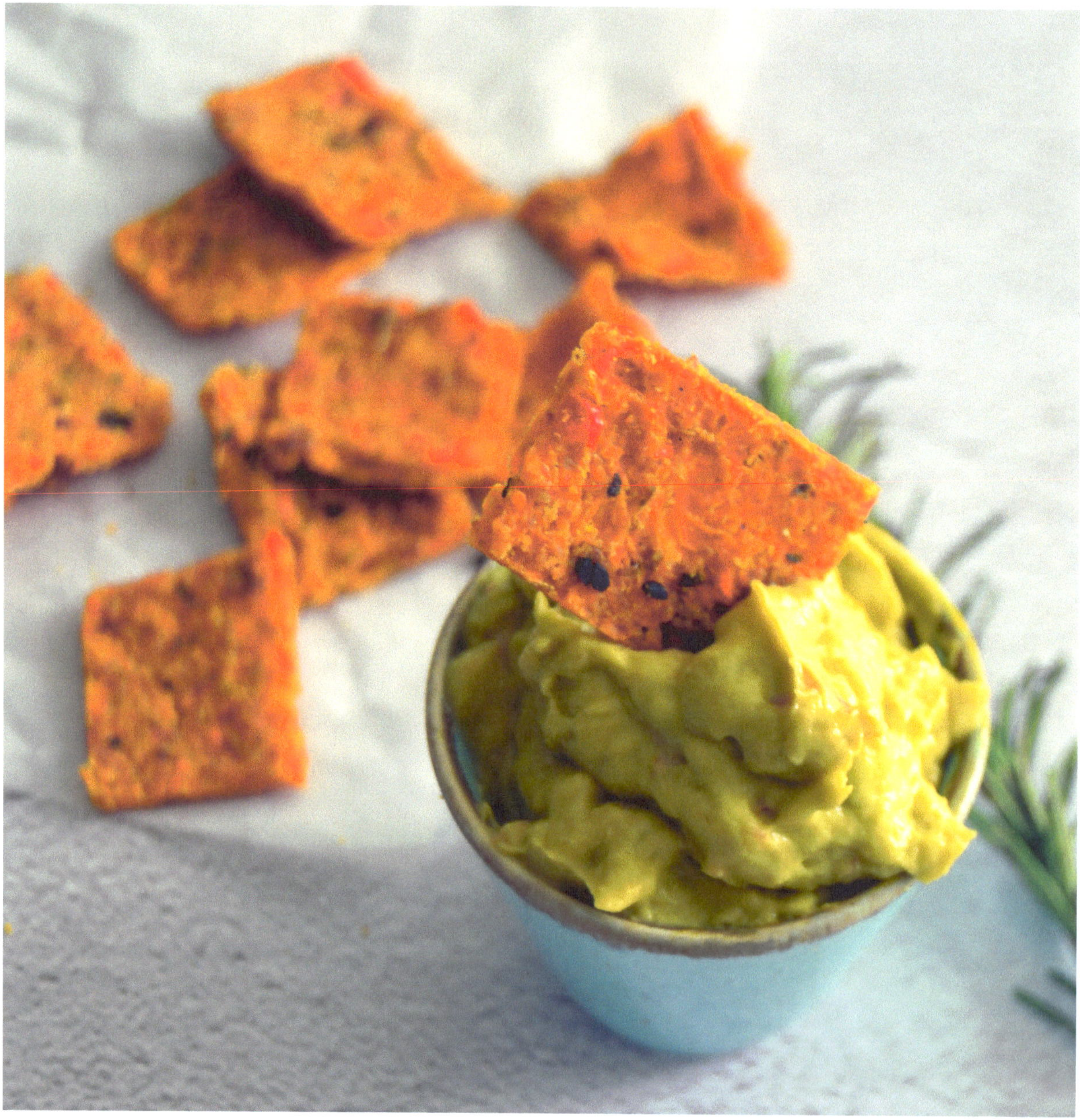

PUMPKIN TURMERIC CRACKERS

Yield: 3-4 person

Ingredients

40 g yellow capriscum
145 g pumpkins
1/2 tsp onion powder
1 tsp garlic powder
1 tsp salt
1 tbsp coconut oil
1 tbsp lemon juice
1 tsp turmeric
4 tbsp water
1 tbsp maple syrup
1/4 tsp cayenne
2 tbsp almond meal
2 tbsp ground golden flaxseeds

In a small bowl add the water and ground flax, let them rest for 10 minutes.

Add the rest of the ingredients into the food processor and mix until you get dough consistency. Then add the flax mixture, blend again.

Remove dough from the food processor. Make a ball with your hands. Place the ball between two sheets of parchment paper and roll out with a rolling pin as thin as possible, without breaking any of the edges.

Put the rolled out dough on a baking sheet and use a pizza cutter to make scores in the crackers for later.

Dehydrate for about 8 hours and then flip. Bake another 2 hours or until crisp on both sides as you need. Enjoy alone or dip in guacamole sauce.

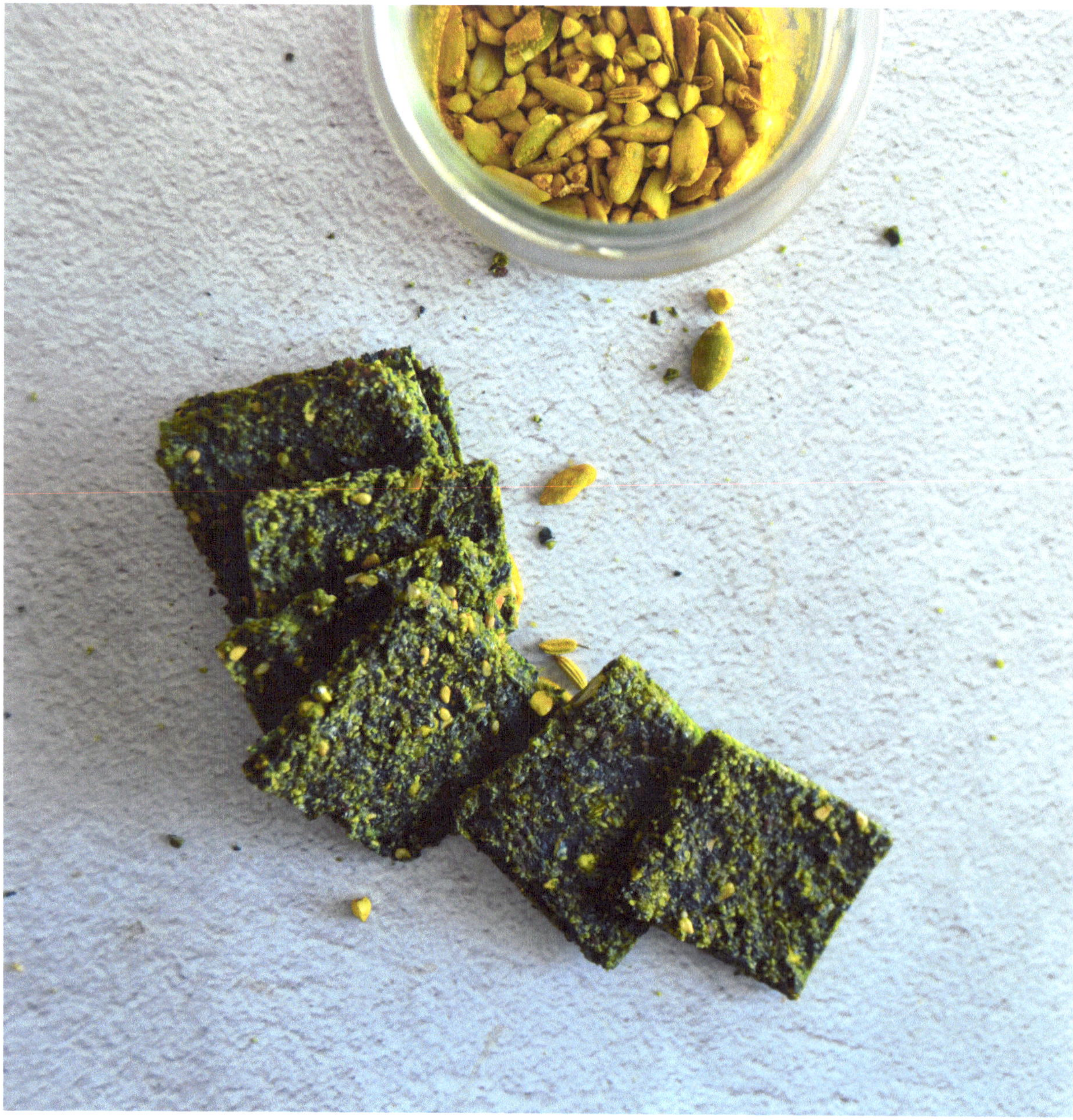

SPINACH SAUERKRAUT CRACKERS

Yield: 4 person

Ingredients

400 g spinach puree
1 tsp onion powder
1/2 tsp garlic powder
1 tbsp maple syrup
1 tsp salt
2 tbsp lemon juice
4 tbsp water
1 cup sprouted pea flour (or use almond flour)
3 tbsp ground flaxseed
2 tsp sauerkraut spices (or use 2 tbsp pickled sauerkraut finely chopped)
2 tbsp sesame seeds

In a small bowl add water and ground flax, let them rest for 10 minutes.

Add all remaning ingredients into the food processor and mix until get dough consistency.

Then add flax mix, blend again. Remove dough from the food processor.

Make a ball with your hands.
Place the ball between two sheets of parchment and roll out with a rolling pin as thin as possible, without breaking any of the edges.

Put the rolled out dough on a baking sheet and cut into squares.
Dehydrate for about 8 hours and then flip.
Bake another 2 hours or until crisp on both sides if you need.

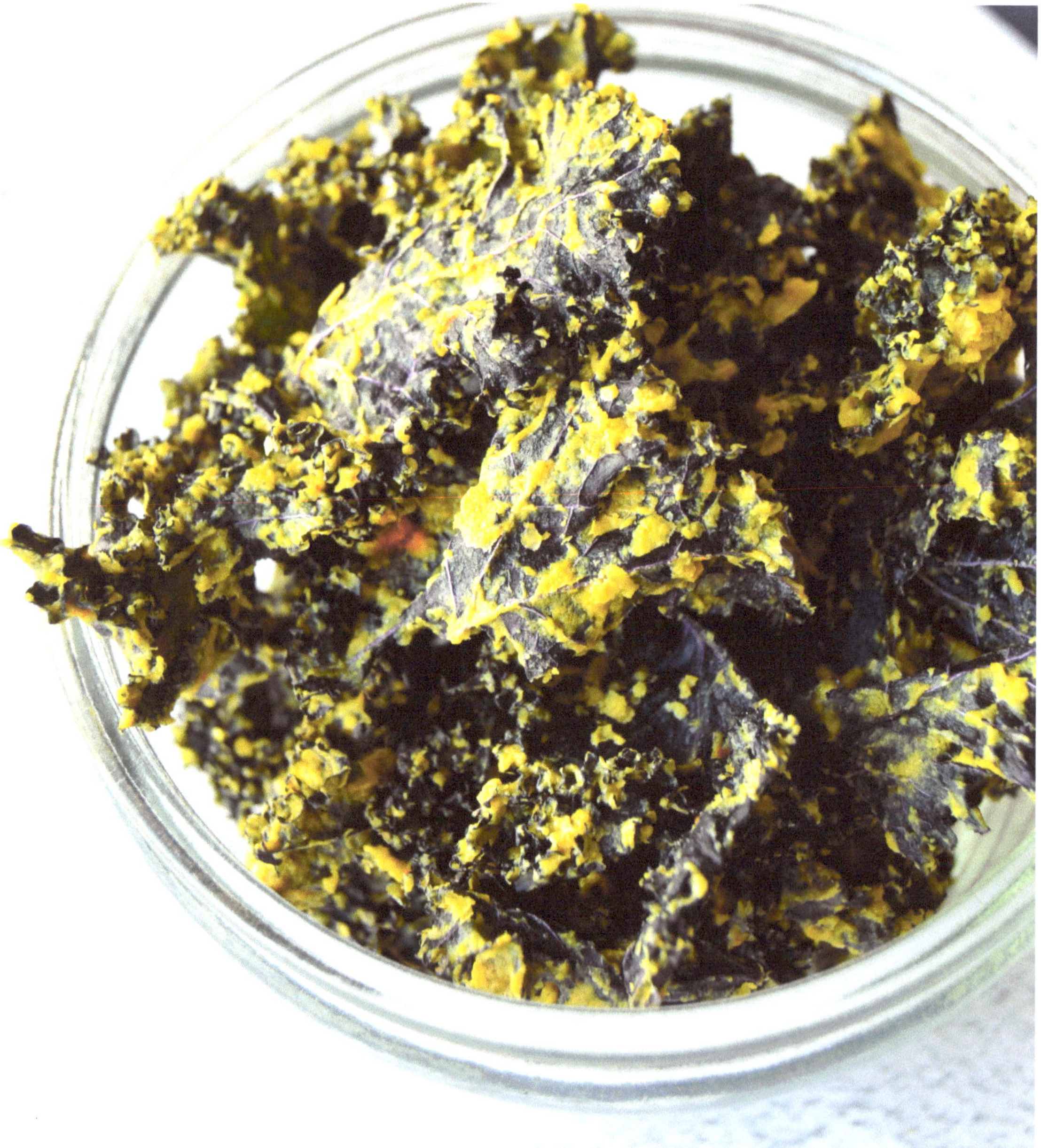

DEHYDRATED KALE CHIPS WITH TURMERIC CHEESE SAUCE

Yield: 2-4 person

Ingredients

300 g kale
1/2 cup sunflower seeds
3-4 tbsp water
3 tbsp nutritional yeast
1 tsp salt
Juice of whole lemon
1 tsp garlic powder
1/2 tsp turmeric

First wash, de-stem and rip the kale into your desired "chip size" pieces. Drain and place in a large bowl.

Wash and strain your sunflower seeds, transfer to blendtec or a high speed blender.

Add the rest of the ingredients, blend well until you get smooth sauce.

Pour mixture over the kale pieces. Massage for 4-5 minutes with your hands.

Dehydrate for about 3-4 hours or more at 42°C in excalibur dehydrator until completely crispy. When the chips are dry and crispy, remove and enjoy!

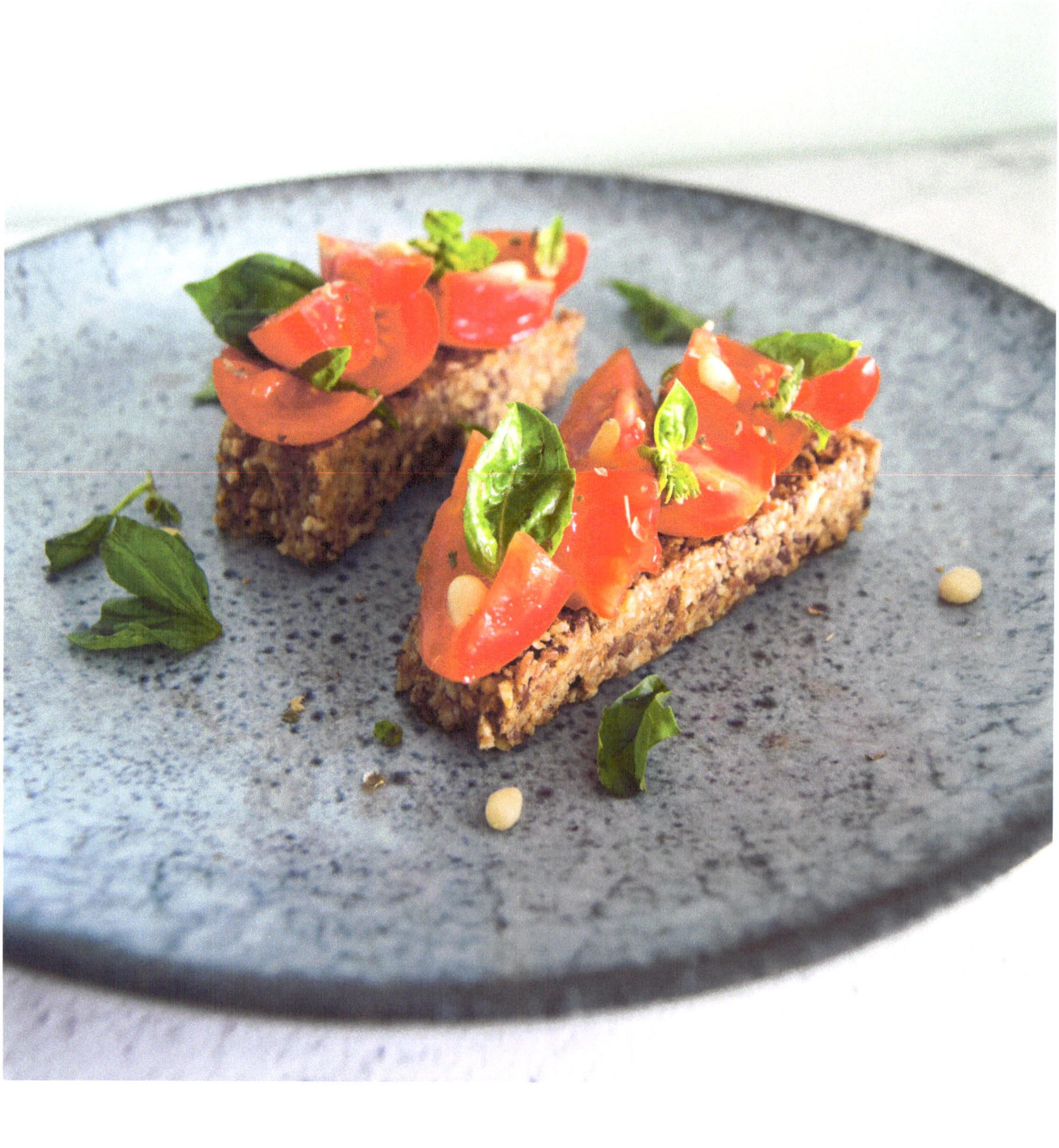

BRUSCHETTA

Yield: 6-8 slices

Ingredients

100 g sprouted buckwheat groats
100 g zucchini
35 g flaxseed grounded
2 tsp white miso paste
1 tsp salt
1 cup water
80 g almond butter
1 tbsp chopped onions
2 garlic cloves minced
2 tbsp nutritional yeast
1 tsp coconut vinegar
2 tbsp coconut nectar syrup
2 tbsp cold press grapeseed oil
2 tbsp psyllium husk powder
35 g coconut flour
60 g hazelnut flour
Fresh Basil & Tomatoes to serve

In a large jar, blend, flax seeds, miso, salt and water. Close the lid of the jar and let it ferment in the dehydrator at 33 C for 10-12 hours.
Place sprouted and drained buckwheat in a high speed blender, add fermented mixture and the rest of the ingredients expect psyllium husk powder and tomato and basil. 3. 3. Process for few minutes until combined well.
Remove mixture from the blender, transfer to a large bowl. Add the psyllium husk and knead well with your hands until combined well.
Let it sit for few minutes until firm up and psyllium absorbs the water.
Form the dough into a log or desired shape and dehydrate on a nonstick sheet for 8-12 hours at 42°C.
Remove from nonstick sheet and dry again for the next 8-hours.
Slice the bread using a very sharp knife and dehydrate again to dry the inside, about 2-3 hours.
Once done, top with halved cherry tomatoes and fresh basil. Drizzle extra virgin olive oil if desired, enjoy!

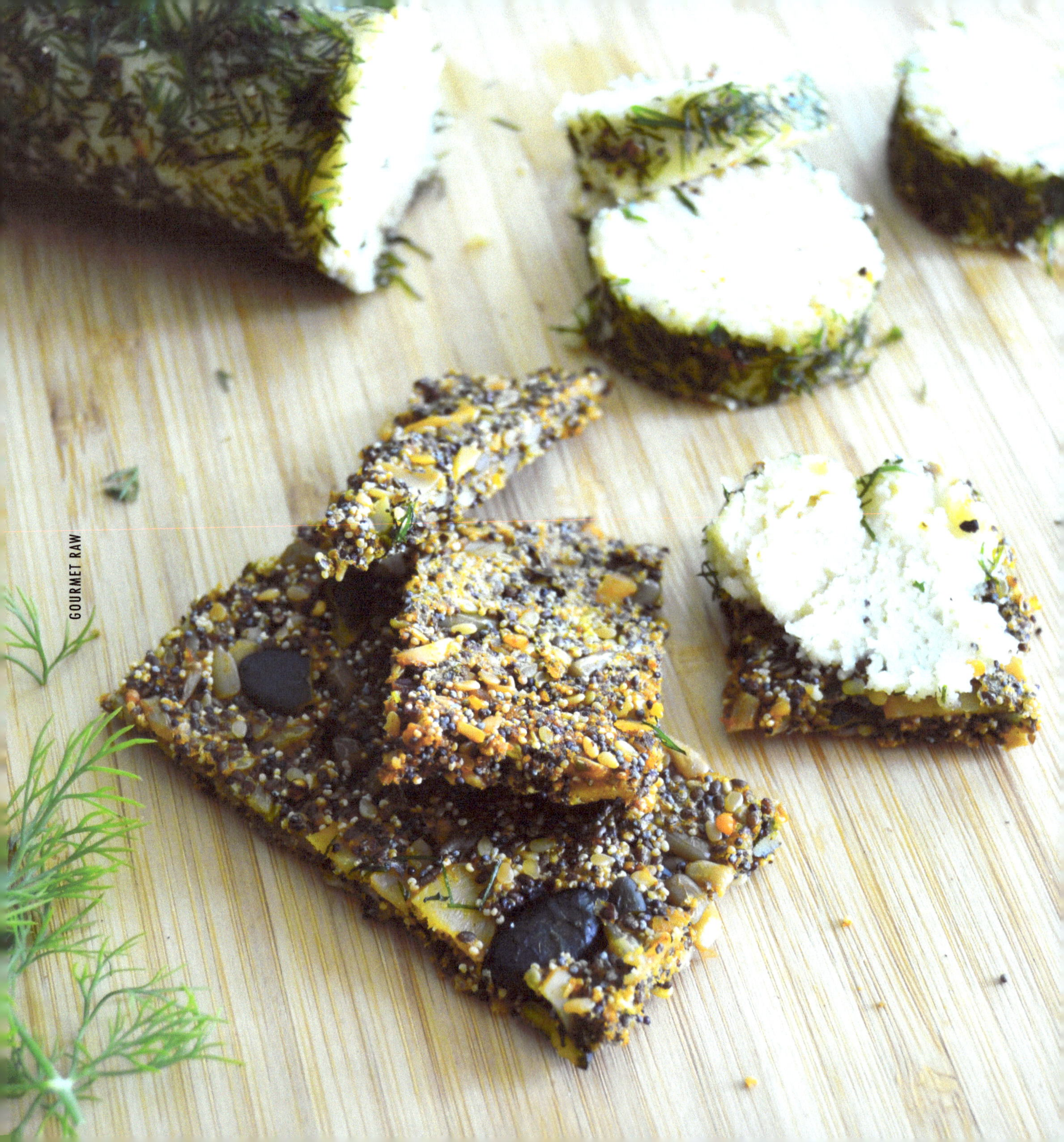

MACADAMIA CHEESE

Nuts contain levels of phytic acid equal to or higher than those of grains. When we ferment the nuts, phytates are eliminated. Soaking nuts makes the food more digestible.

Yield: 6

Ingredients

220 g raw macadamia nuts
4 g acidophilus probiotic
1/3 cup filtered water
2 tbsp nutritional yeast
2 tbsp lemon juice
1/4 tsp sea salt
1/2 bunch fresh dill

Place nuts in a jar. Cover with filtered warm water and close the jar. Let it rest in the room at least 1 hour. Then place in the fridge for 6 hours.This process will activate the nuts and also yields a neutral nut flavor.
Set 6 tablespoons water from the soaked nuts aside. Strain and rise nuts. Place nuts and 6 tablespoons water into the food processor. Mix on high speed until silky smooth. If you are using probiotic powder then dissolve it in a little water.
Then transfer into the food processor. Mix well. Transfer nut mixture into a nut milk bag. Gather up the ends to create a ball. Wrap the ends and squeeze out any excess moisture.
Place cheese in the dehydrator at 30 degrees for about 20-24 hours to let it ferment.
House with an average temperature of 25-30°C for 24 hours.

Once the fermentation time is up, open the cheesecloth and observe your nut cheese very carefully. You will probably notice that a yellowish crust has formed on top. That is totally normal. The inside of the nut cheese should be spongy. If there is pink or bluish spots, it indicates the presence of mold; throw away the cheese and restart. If everything is ok, transfer cheese from its cloth to a bowl and stir in nutritional yeast, garlic, lemon juice and salt. At this point you could add in other flavors whatever you like. If you like a stronger cheese flavor, add a bit more nutritional yeast. Form a log or ball on a piece of parchment paper and place in the fridge for overnight.

Last step is rolling in a salty herby mixture. On a flat surface, spread out fresh dill or your herbs and sprinkle on some salt. Take your cheese and give it a good roll in the herbs. Place in the fridge at least 3 days to age the your cheese. If you like a softer cheese, you can use cashews instead of macadamia nuts, or a mix of both nuts. In that case, you will need less than ½ cup of water, because cashews are creamier to blend.

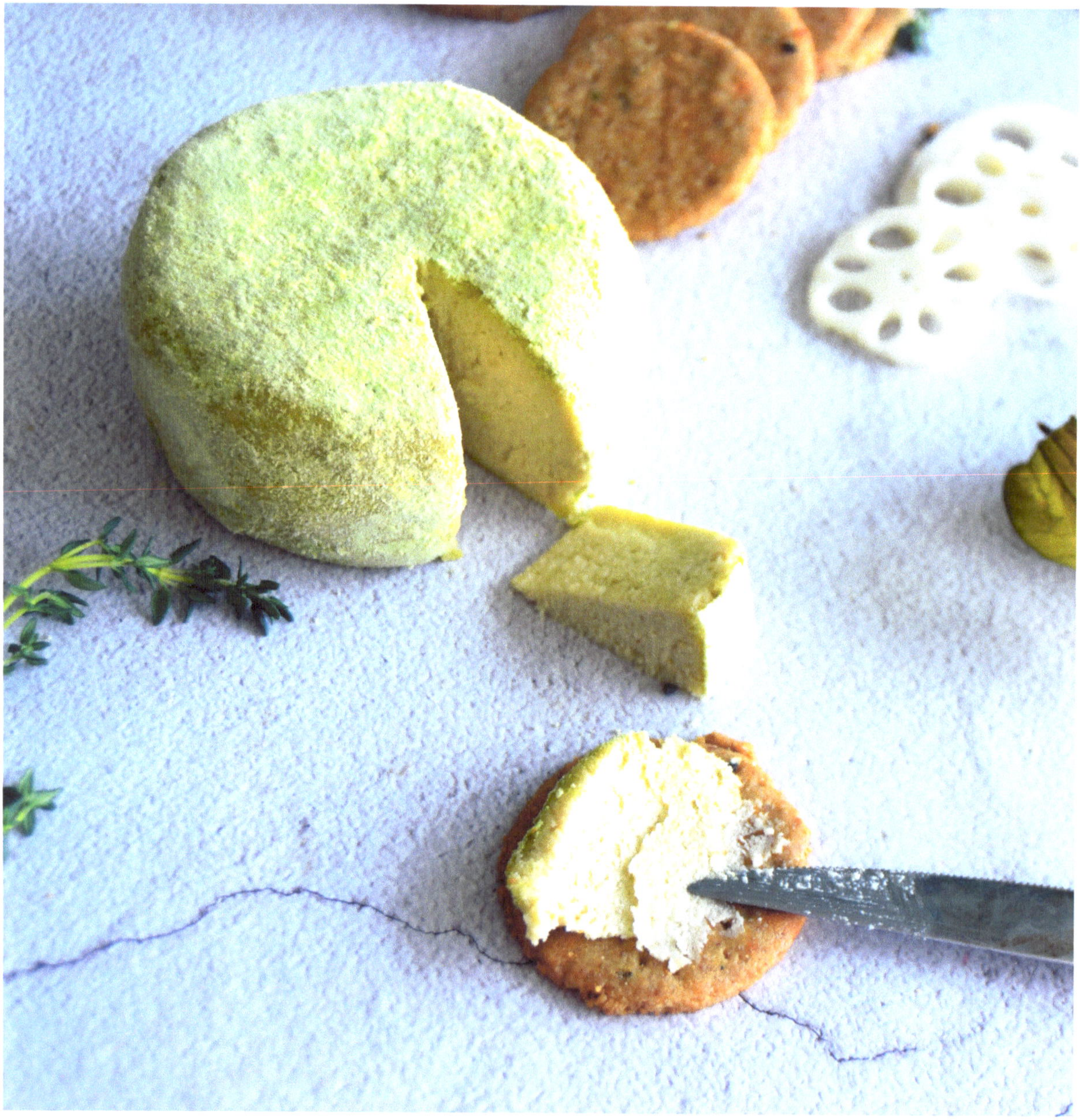

AGED WASABI CASHEW CHEESE

Yield: 4-6 person

Ingredients

200 g raw cashews soaked
2 g acidophilus probiotic
1 tbsp sweet white miso
1/3 cup filtered water
3 tbsp nutritional yeast
2 tbsp lemon juice
1/2 tsp sea salt
2 tbsp wasabi powder + more for coating

Place the cashews in the bowl of a blender or food processor. Add the filtered water, sweet white miso, lemon juice, salt, wasabi and nutritional yeast. Blend on high speed, scraping down the sides from time to time, until you get a very smooth and thick mixture.
Add the probiotic to the blender and blend on high speed for another 10-15 seconds. The cashew cream should be smooth but thick. If needed, add 1 tablespoon of water at a time until smooth.
Transfer the mixture to a clean mixing bowl and cover with plastic film to touch. This will prevent the top from drying. Let sit at room temperature for at least 12 hours. This step is important to let the cheese ferment.
The next day, place the bowl in the refrigerator for about 3-4 hours. The cashew cream will slighty firm up, making it easier to work with.

Cut strips of parchment paper and lay them in 2 small springform pans. You want to cover the sides and bottom of the springform pans, you can also use plastic film if you prefer.
Fill each pan with the mixture and press it down using plastic film so it doesn't stick to your hands. Place the springform pans in the refrigerator, or at a temperature of 10°C.
The next day, carefully remove the cheeses from the springform pans and sprinkle about 1/4 tsp of salt and wasabi over the top of each cheese, rub with your finger to evenly distribute. Flip the cheeses and sprinkle the bottom and sides with more salt and wasabi powder.
Place the cheeses on a plate lined with parchment paper in your refrigerator. The next day, your cheeses will have lost some water. Pat them dry with a paper towel if they are too wet, and replace the parchment paper with a new one. Age the cheeses at 10°C for the next two weeks and flip them every 2-3 days. Do not store the cheeses at a temperature higher than 12°C or they could turn bad.
During the first week, the cheeses will be very soft but as they age they will become firmer. If you see some mold appearing, just scrape it off and re-salt the area.

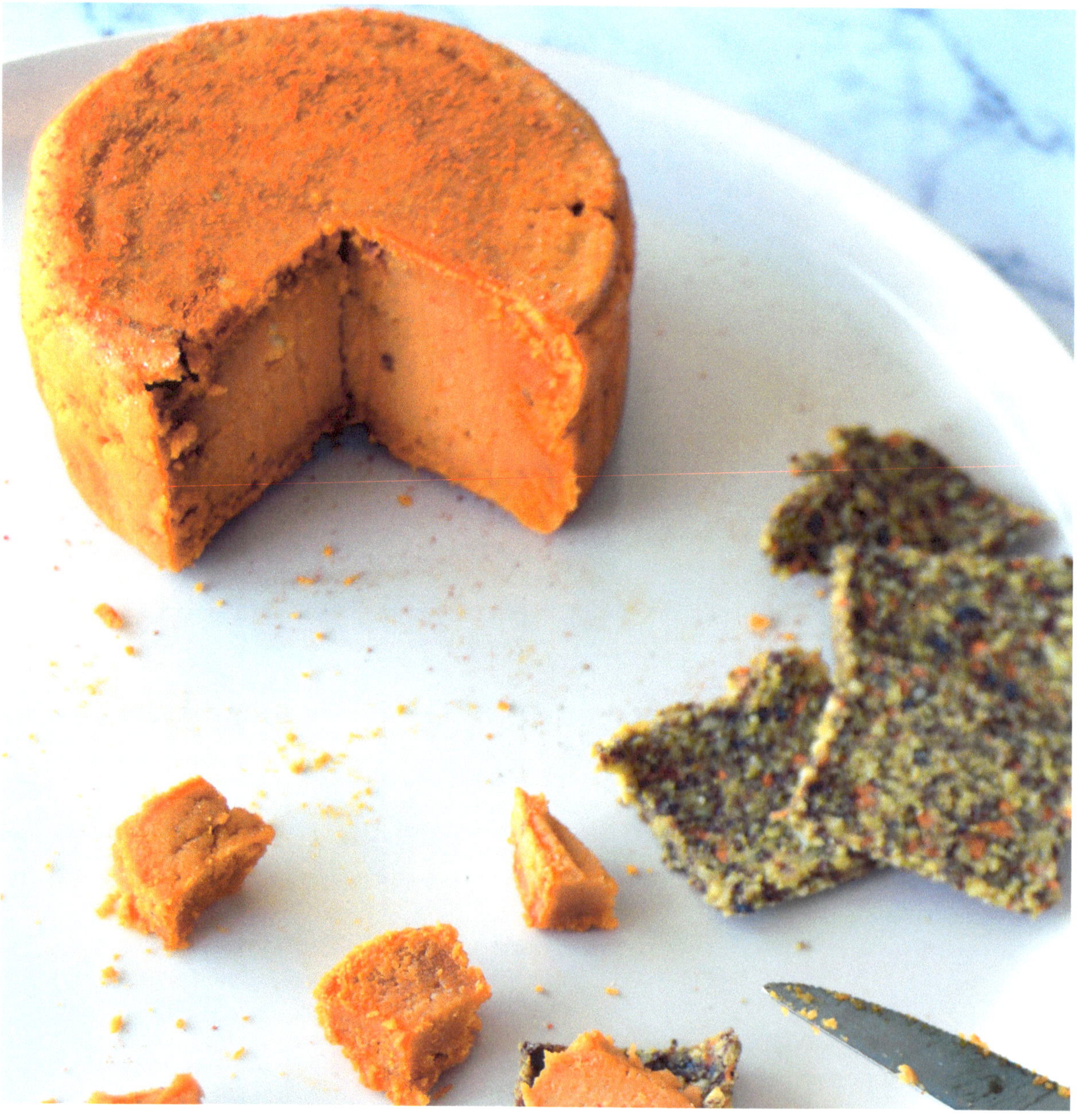

AGED SUNFLOWER SEED TOMATO CHEESE

Yield: 4-6 person

Ingredients

140 g sunflower seeds soaked
100 g almonds peeled soaked
5 g acidophilus probiotic
1/4 cup filtered water as needed
4 tbsp nutritional yeast
8 pieces sundried tomatoes
2 tbsp lemon juice
2 tsp pink himalayan salt
2 tbsp paprika for coating

Soak the sunflower seeds and almonds together in slightly warm water for 3-4 hours, then rinse and place in the food processor.

Add the rest of the ingredients.

Blend on high speed, scraping down the sides from time to time until you get smooth texture. In this period if you need, add more water but avoid adding too much. The consistency should not be too soft.

Transfer the your mixture into a cheesecloth and pull it tight. Add a weight above it and let sit at dehydrator for about 24 hours. This step is important to start the fermentation of the mixture and drain possible excess water.

The next day, the mixture should have a slightly sour, lemony taste, like fresh cream cheese. Transfer to a spring pan, cover with plastic film to touch and place in the refrigerator for about 6 hours. After 6 hours, remove the cheese from the springform pans and place it on a plate or small baking sheet lined with parchment paper. Salt both sides with about 1/4 tsp of salt and paprika. Place in the refrigerator for 2 days.

As you can consume the cheese after two days, you can leave more days to age. The cheese will have lost some water day by day. If you will go to age more days, pat it dry with a paper towel if it is too wet, and replace the parchment paper with a new one. Once it reaches to hard texture as you want, use in your dishes.

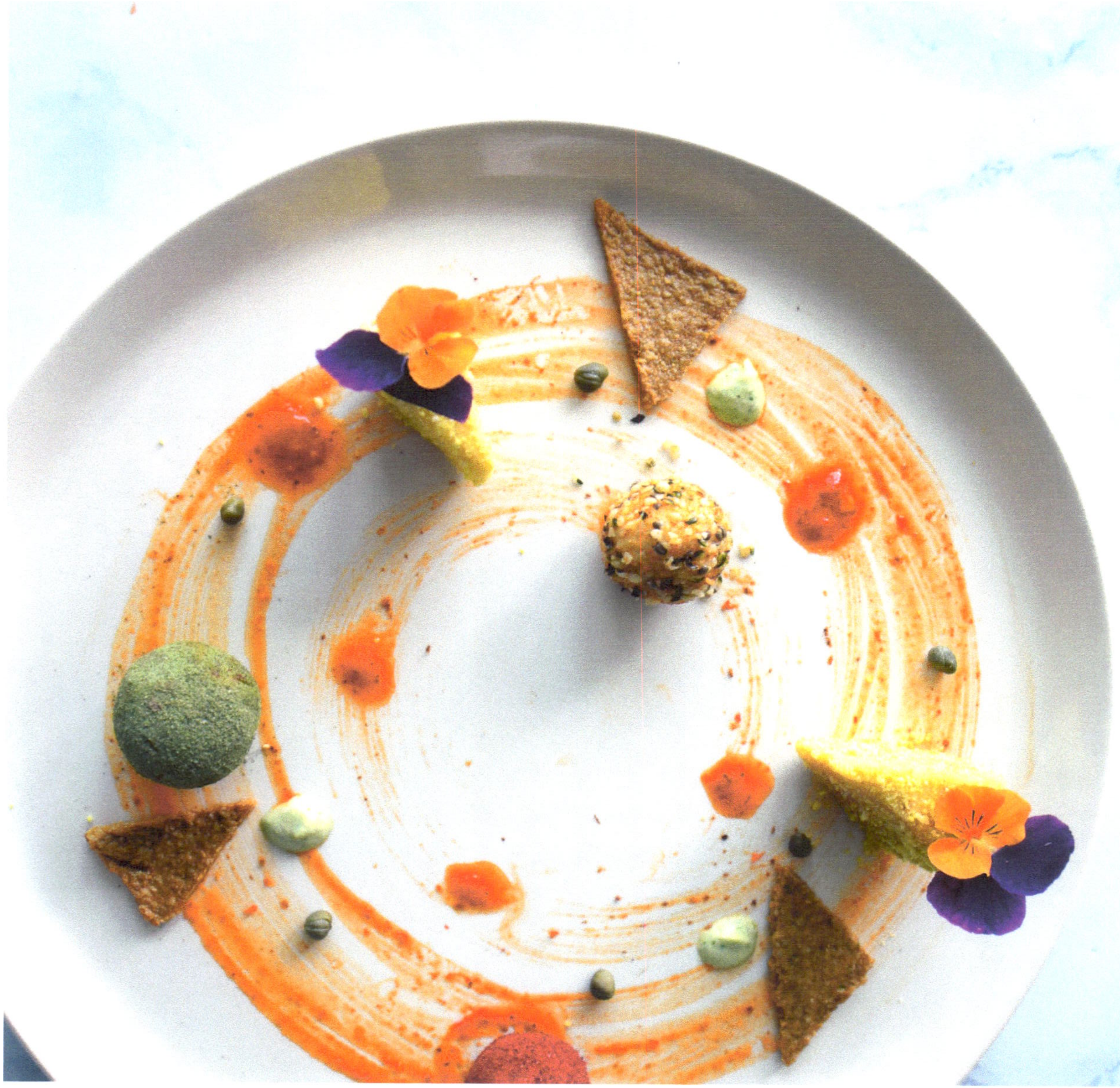

COSMIC NUT CHEESE PLATE

Yield: 4-6 person

Ingredients

Mixed fermented Nut Cheeses (page 61,65)
Rachos (page 39)
Sweet chili sauce (page 17)
Edible flowers
Dehydrated raw beet powder
Raw spinach powder
Rawmesan
Capers
Hemp hearts
Tartar sauce (page 17)
Dried cherries

See nut cheese recipes on page 61, 65 , After fermentation process, when your cheese is ready to eat, scoop a tablespoon, put a dried cherry in the middle, give it a ball shape using your hands. Roll into beet powder. Repeat the process for the rest and make at least 3 ball per plate. Cover with spinach powder, hemp hearts or whatever you want. To make triangle cheese, cut your cheese in triangle using a sharp knife. Dip it in rawmesan, cover completely with rawmesan.

Make your chili and tartar sauce according to recipes on page 17. Chill before plating.

Take a large white plate, using a brush draw a circle with the chili sauce . Then draw a smaller circle in the middle of the large circle.
Place your cheeses in the large circle leaving two fingers space. Place the crackers you cut triangles between cheese balls.

Using a small teaspoon , drop small dots with chili sauce and tartar sauce around the circle. Decorate with capers and edible flowers. Enjoy!

DEHYDRATED PINE NUT CHEESE

Yield: 6-8 person

Ingredients

3 cups pine nuts

3 tbsp lemon juice

2 tbsp nutritional yeast

1 tbsp green onion chopped

1 tsp pink himalayan salt

1 tsp garlic powder

Place all ingredients to the food processor, mix them until chunky. Drop a spoon onto dehydrator sheets . Repeat the process. Dehydrate at 42°C for 5-6 hours or until completely dry on the outside but still tender on the inside. Store in the airtight container in the refrigerator for up to a week.

It is perfect with summer salads like strawberry, asparagus or tabouli. You can also add fresh herbs directly to this recipe!

EASY FRESH CASHEW CHEESE

Yield: 4-6 person

Ingredients

2 cups raw cashews soaked
4 tbsp lemon juice
2 tbsp nutritional yeast
1 tsp pink himalayan salt
1 cup yellow capriscum
1 tsp dried rosemary or fresh rosemary (alternatively you can use fresh dill)

Place yellow capriscum to the blender, add the lemon juice and salt.
Mix on high speed until you get puree. Then add cashew and the rest of the ingredients. Process on high speed until you get smooth mixture.
Place mixture in a glass jar, keep in the refrigerator up to 2-3 days.

You can replace cashews with almonds or macadamia and use red bell pepper in place of yellow one according to your taste.

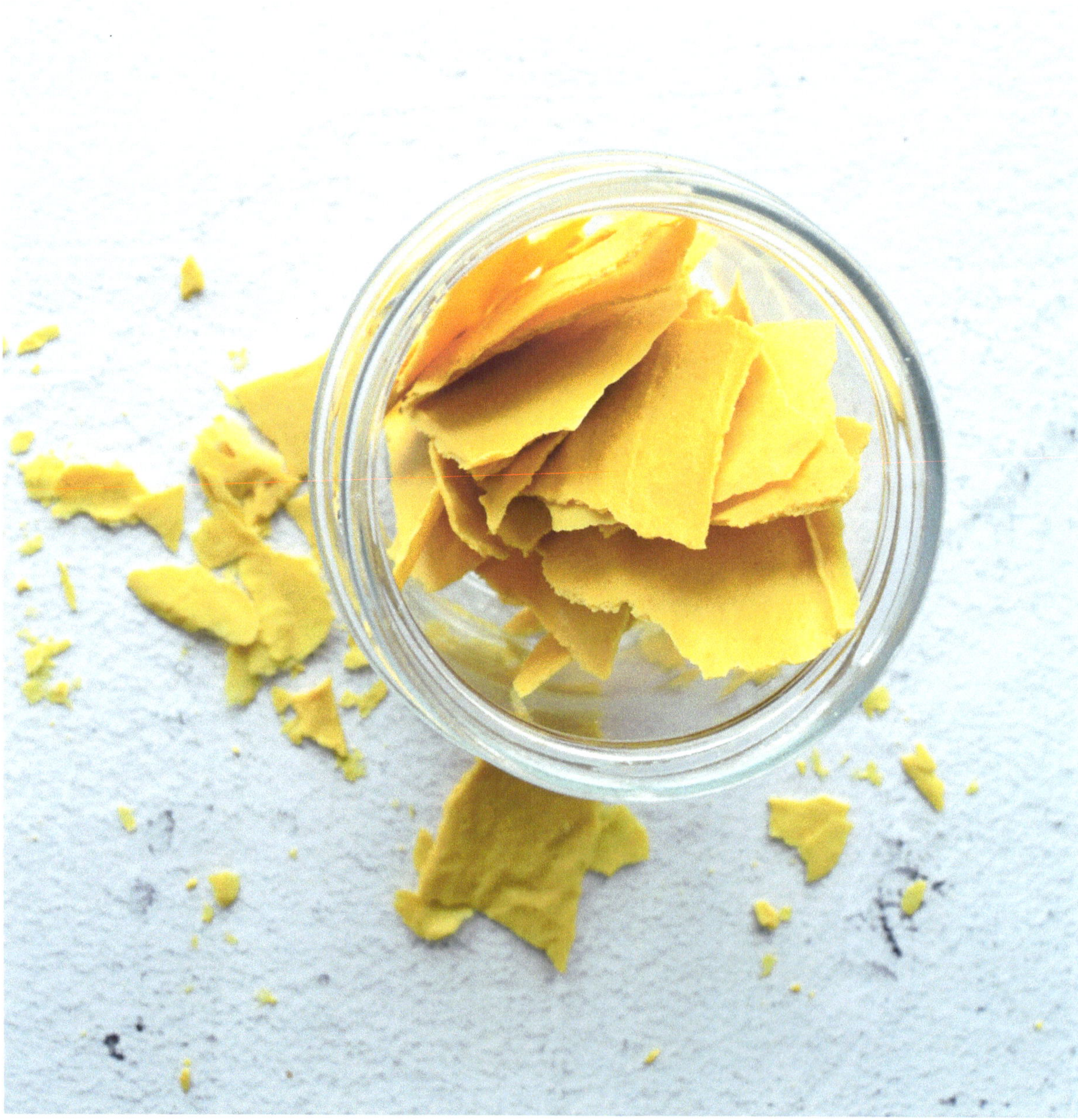

RAWMESAN THINS

Yield: 4 person

Ingredients

140 g sunflower seeds or cashews (alternatively almond and sunflower seeds can be mixed together)
5 tbsp of nutritional yeast
3 tbsp of lemon juice
1 tsp of coconut aminos
1 tbsp of apple cider vinegar
A pinch of turmeric powder
1/8 tsp chili (optional)
1/2 tsp pink himalayan salt or more if you need
1/2 tsp mushroom powder (optional preferably dried porcini, portobello or shiitake)
1/2 tsp garlic powder
5-6 tbsp of water

Soak the nuts in the water for 2-3 hours, then rinse and drain, transfer to the blendtec twister jar.

Add the remaining ingredients to the blender. Mix at high speed until you get a smooth mixture.
Place a non-stick paper to a dehydrator tray. Spread the cheese mixture very thinly using offset spatula.

Bake it in the dehydrator at 42 ° C for about 10-12 hours.

After 6 hours, flip the cheese, transfer to a new parchment paper. Then cook back side of the cheese for another 6 hours.
When your cheese is baked, cut it into small pieces and keep it in the jar. Alternatively you can place it into the food processor and blend until you get powder form and use as parmesan powder for pasta, salad or whatever you want.

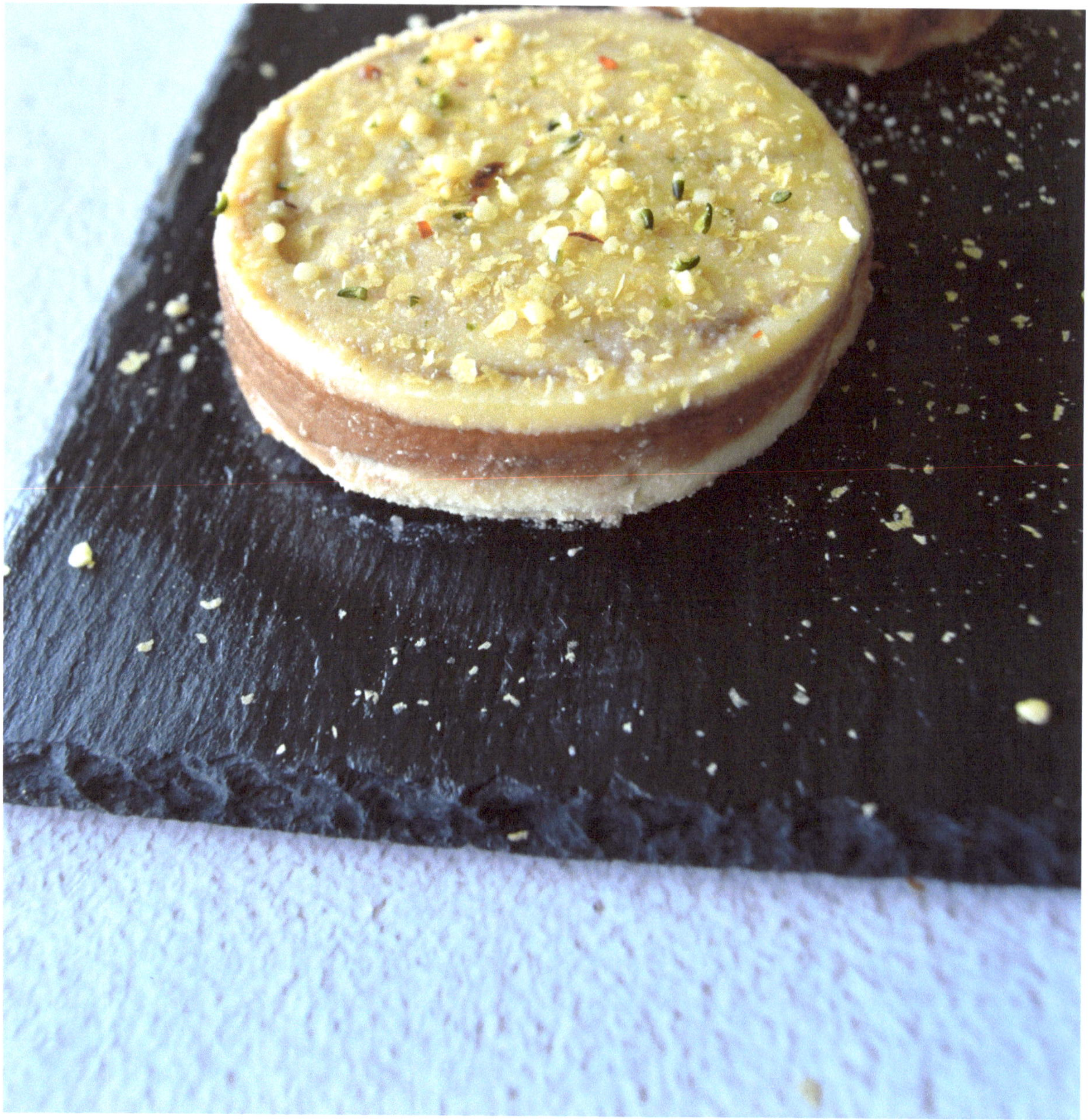

MULLED LAVA SPICED NUT CHEESE

Yield: 6-8 person

Lava Reduction

45 ml icelandic bitter lava
A sachet of Steenbergs mulled wine spices (or 1 tbsp blend of cinnamon, clove, nutmeg, ginger and coriander)
2 tbsp maple or coconut nectar
200 ml water
1 tbsp fresh orange juice

Nut Cheese

200 g raw cashews soaked
60 ml water
1 probiotic capsule
1/2 tsp smoked sea salt
2 tbsp nutritional yeast
2 tbsp lemon Juice
1 cup lava reduction

To make lava reduction, place all the lava reduction ingredients in a saucepan, put a thermometer in the pan and slowly heat maximum at 42°C. Mixing slowly cook for 30-35 minutes than strain. Remove sachet and keep the liquid. Continue to heat liquid over medium heat for 10 minutes. Transfer in a glass jar. Set aside.

Soak and rinse your cashews, transfer to a high speed blender, add the probiotic and water. Blend until smooth.

Place mixture in a glass jar, cover with cheesecloth. Let it sit at room temperature for at least 24 hours to culture. Once fermentation is done, open jar, add smoked salt or just salt, nutritional yeast and lemon juice. Mix using a wooden spoon well. Transfer mixture to a round mold. Place in the freezer for 1-1,5 hours or until firm.

Place cheese wheels in the bowls with mulled lava spice. Cover with plastic wrap. Refrigerate for 24 hours.
Then remove from the lava, place on a plate, put the fridge for additional 2 hours before consuming.

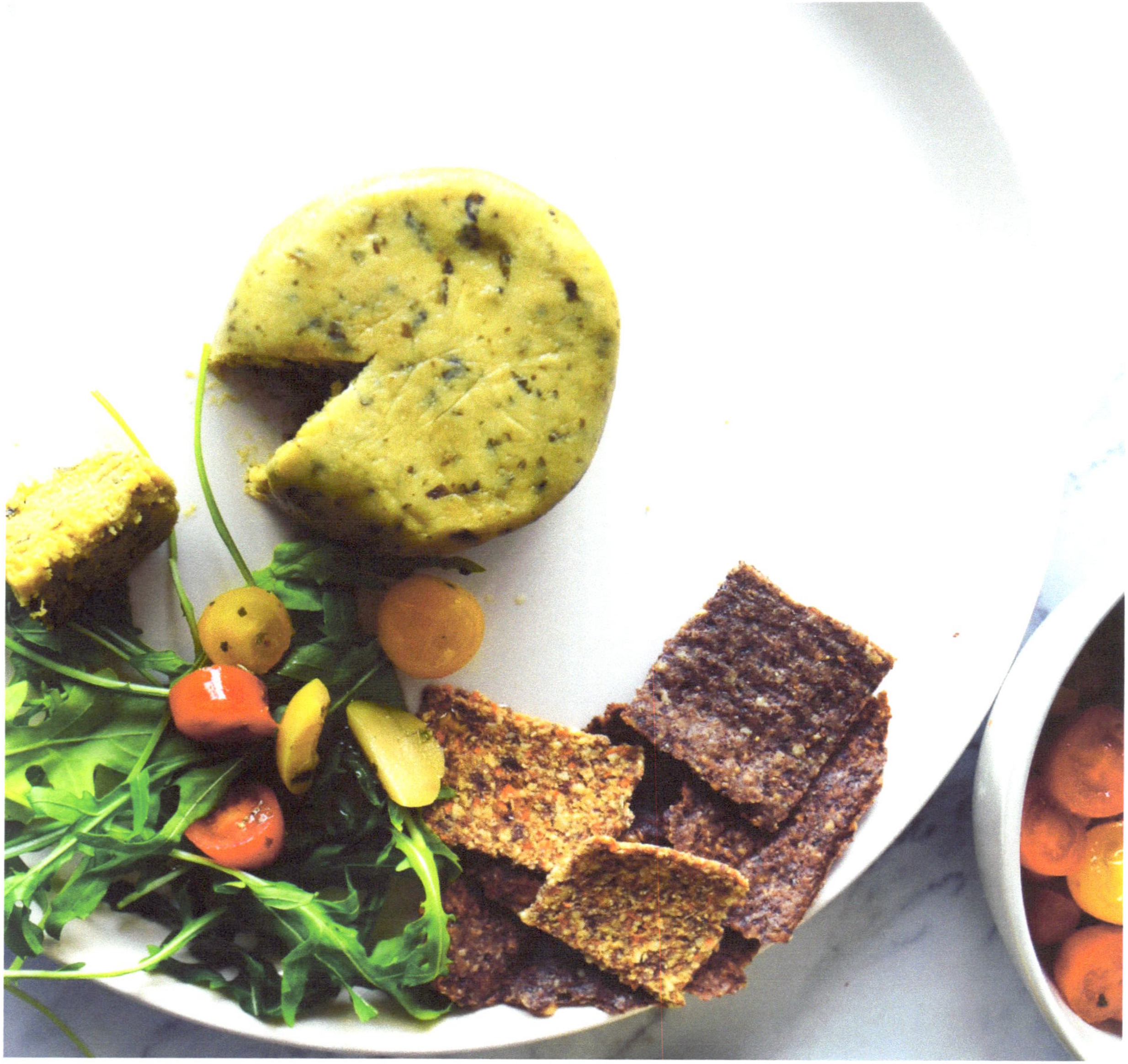

AGED BASIL NUT CHEESE

Yield: 4 person

Ingredients

200 g raw cashew nuts
4 g probiotic
2-3 tbsp filtered water as needed
2 tbsp nutritional yeast
20 g fresh basil
2 tbsp lemon juice
2 tsp pink himalayan salt
1 tbsp olive oil

Soak cashews overnight, then drain and place in the food processor. Add nutritional yeast, lemon juice, basil, salt, olive oil, probiotic and filtered water. Blend on high speed, scraping down the sides from time to time until you get smooth texture. In this period if you need, add more water but avoid adding too much. The consistency should not be too soft.

Transfer the your mixture into a cheesecloth and pull it tight. Add a weight above it and let sit at dehydrator for about 24 hours.. This step is important to start thea fermentation of the cashew cream and drain possible excess water.

The next day, the mixture should have a slightly sour, lemony taste, like fresh cream cheese. Transfer to spring bowl, cover with plastic film to touch and place in the refrigerator for about 6 hours. The goal is to prevent the cheese from sticking to the metal. After 6 hours, remove the cheese from the springform pans and place it on a plate or small baking sheet lined with parchment paper. Salt both sides with about 1/4 tsp of salt. Do the same for the sides. place in the refrigerator for 2 days. Then serve with your raw crackers and salad.

COLOR YOUR NUT CHEESES

Just add little amount of natural coloring plants and fruits to make your cheeses colorful. In order to avoid lose of color, always add after the fermentation process.

Pink: strawberries, raspberries, beets, lingonberries

Orange: carrots, paprika, sweet potato, tomato

Yellow: saffron, turmeric

Green: matcha, spinach, swiss chard, collard greens, moringa

Blue: red cabbage + baking soda, butterfly pea powder, blue spirulina

Purple: blueberries, blackberries, black grapes, purple potato

Black: activated charcoal

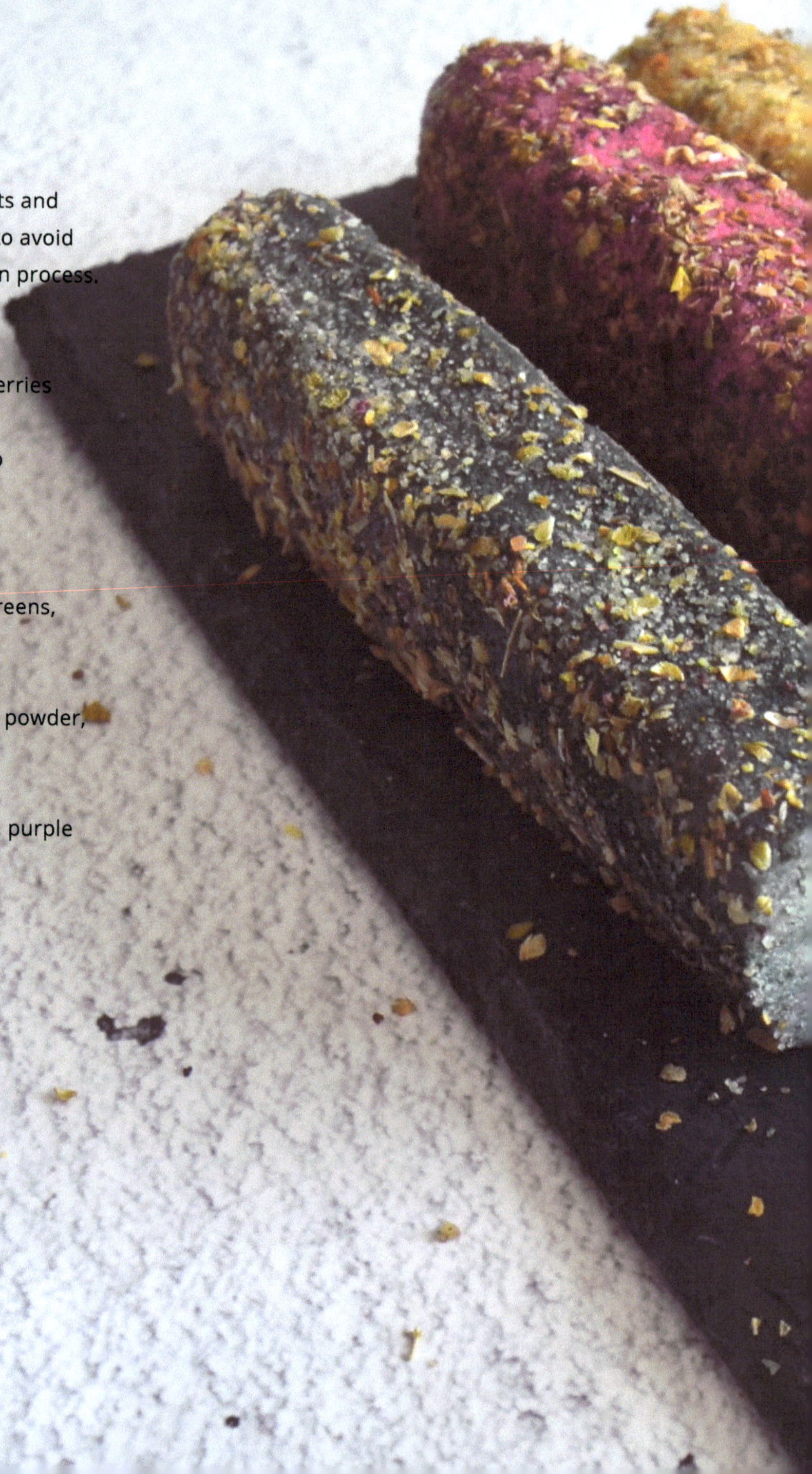

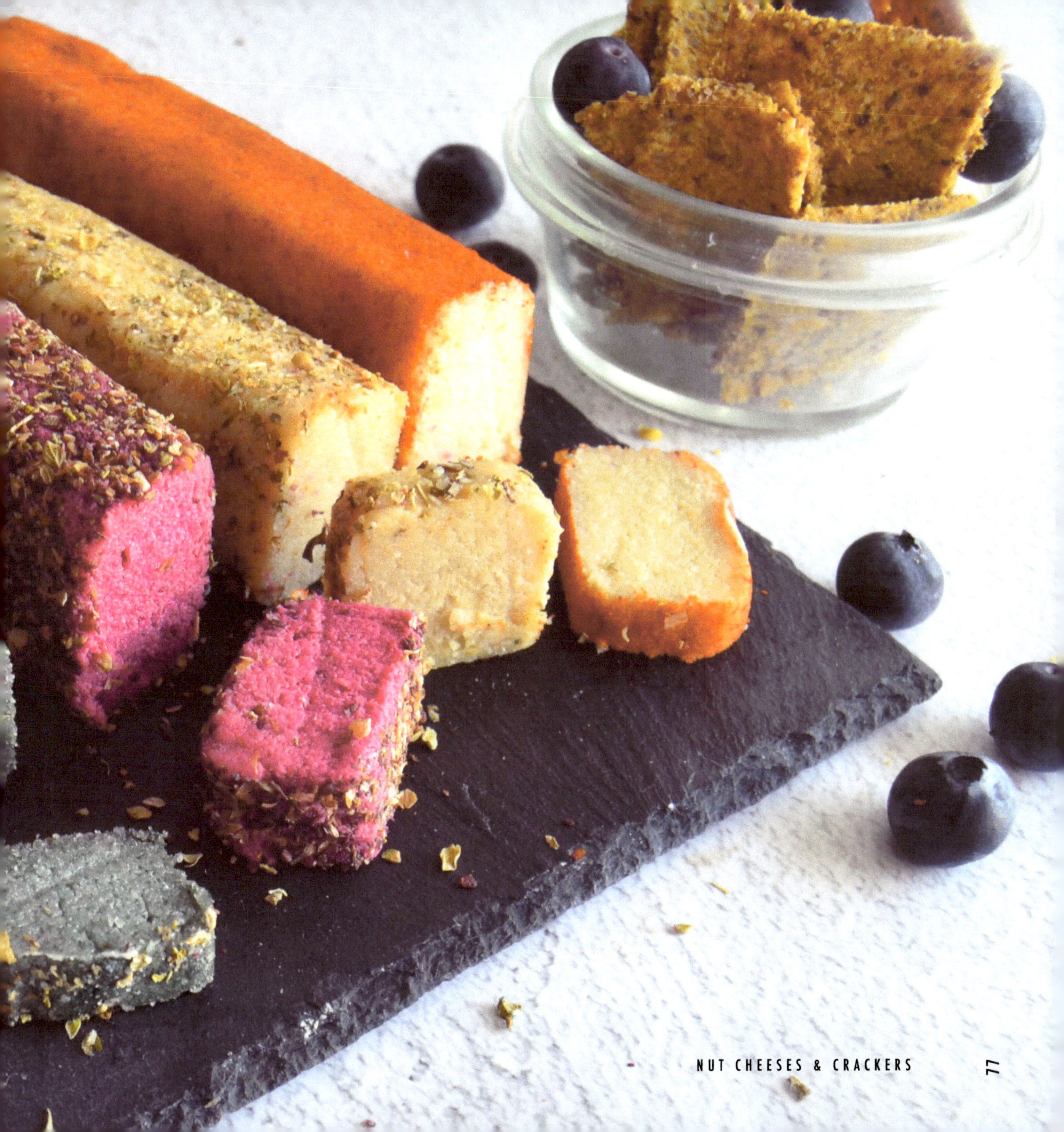

"IF YOU CAN CONTROL WHAT YOU EAT, YOU CAN CONTROL ANYTHING"

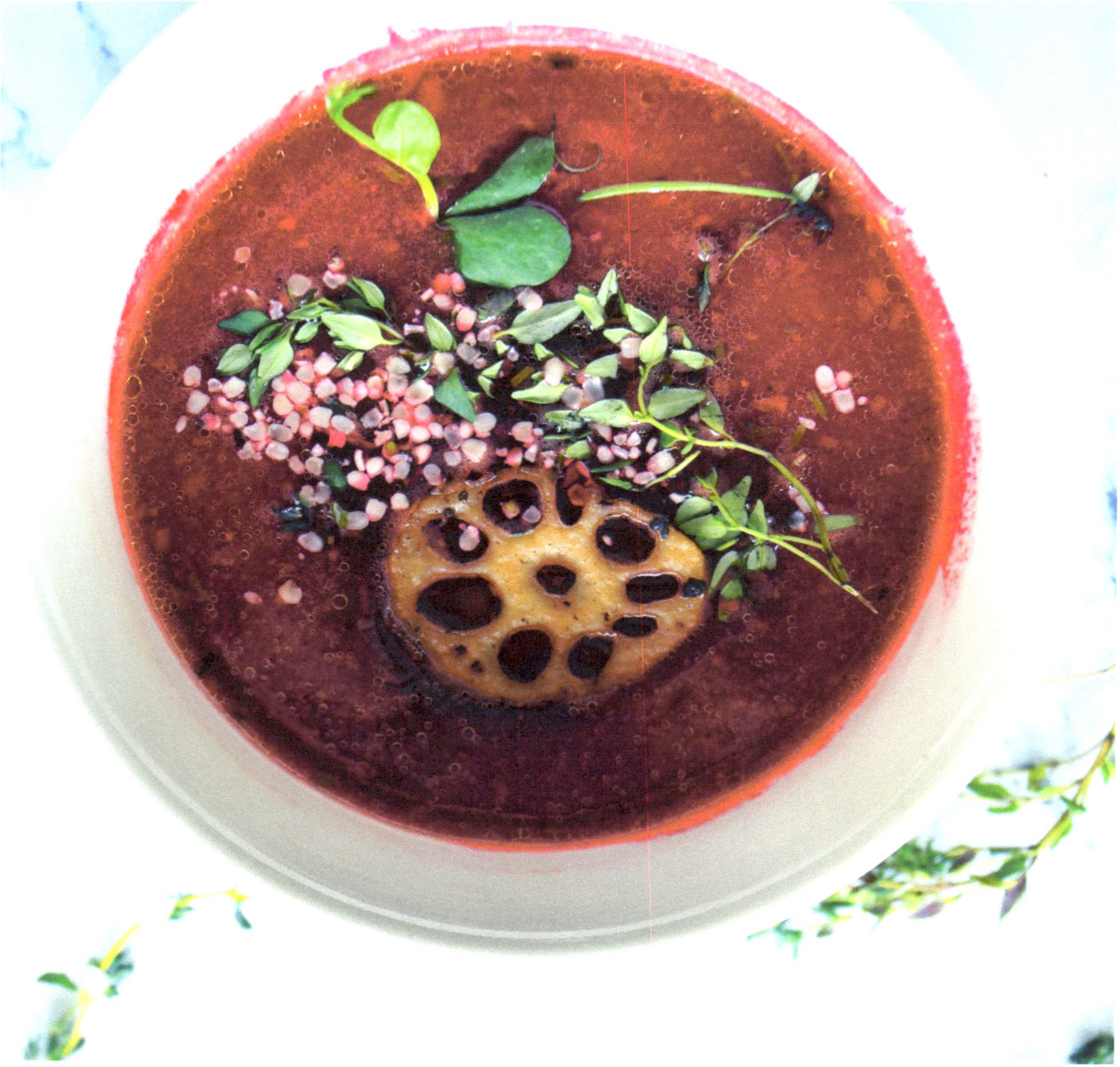

IF A LOTUS COULD SPEAK SOUP

Yield: 2 person

Ingredients

1 cup tomatoes
1 small beetroot
2 cups filtered water
1 tsp pink himalayan salt
2 tbsp lemon juice
1 tbsp olive oil
2-3 springs of fresh thyme to serve
2-3 tbsp hemp hearts to serve
Sprouted pea to serve
Lotus roots to serve

Wash and drain your tomatoes and beetroot. Place in a food processor, add filtered water, olive oil, lemon and salt. Mix on high speed until smooth. Taste your soup if you need add more salt.

Cut lotus roots into thin slices. Marinate in coconut aminos for 2-3 hours or just add plain to your soup.

Wash and chop your fresh thyme and sprouted peas. Set aside.

Divide the soup between two bowls, place in the dehydrator and heat at 42°C for 4-5 hours. Then remove from the dehydrator, add sprouted pea, fresh thyme lotus roots and hemp hearts on top. Serve!

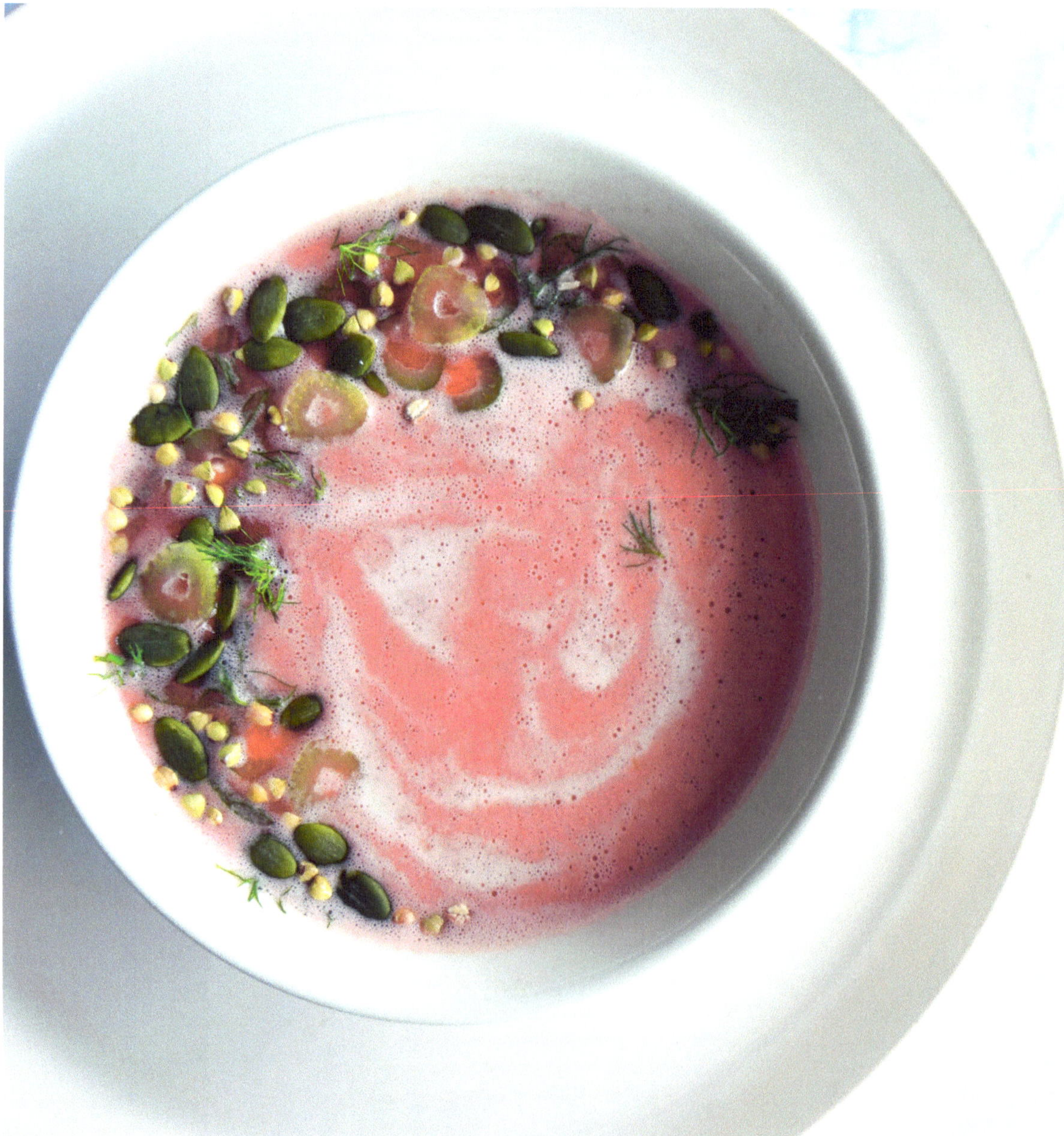

BACHELOR CAULIFLOWER SOUP

Yield: 2 person

Ingredients

200 g cauliflower florets
1 small beetroot
2 tbsp olive oil
3 tbsp lemon juice
2 tbsp finely diced shallot
1 tsp pink himalayan salt
250 ml filtered water
100 ml oat milk

Toppings

Fennel stalks and fronds
Buckinis
Pumpkin seeds
Oat milk

Place all the soup ingredient into your blenders, process on high speed until completely smooth.

Wash your fennel. Finely slice. Set aside.

If you prefer, strain your soup using a cheesecloth or consume as it is. Pour your soup between the bowls.
Decorate with toppings.
Drizzle extra virgin olive oil and blended oat milk foam if desired. Chill and Serve cold!

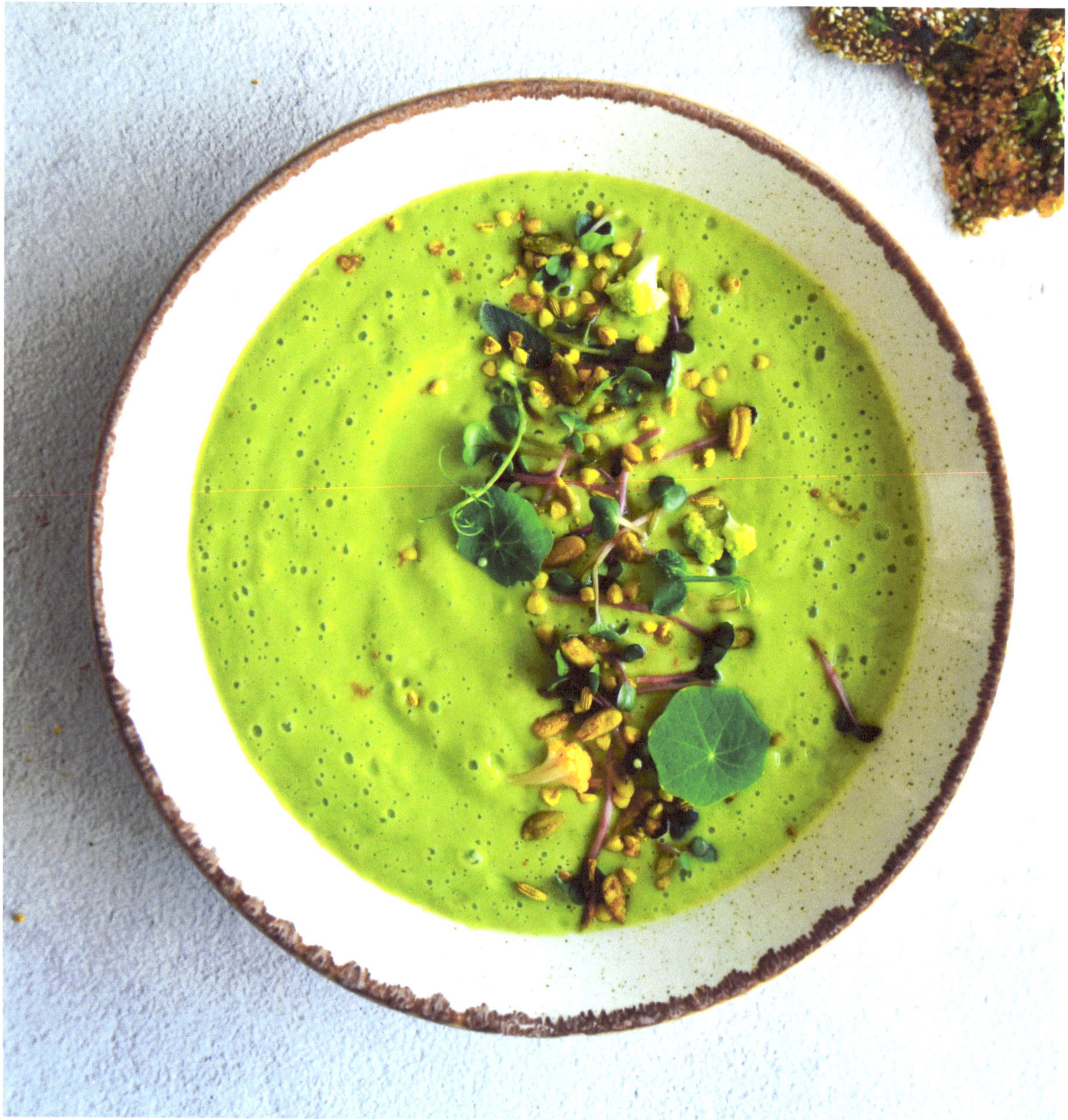

AVOCADO CUCUMBER GAZPACHO

Yield: 2 person

Ingredients

1 medium avocado
2 medium cucumber
1-2 tbsp plant milk or water
1 tbsp white wine vinegar
2 tbsp lemon juice
2 tbsp finely chopped shallot
A pinch of pink himalayan salt

Toppings

Buckini
Cauliflower florets
Sunflower seeds with curry powder
Nasturtium leaves
Zero waste celery crackers to serve

Peel your avocado, remove the seed. Throw in the blender, add all remaining ingredients, process on high speed until completely smooth. Add more plant milk or water if you need until reach the desired consistency.

Pour your soup in the bowls. Garnish with toppings if desired. Chill and Serve cold!

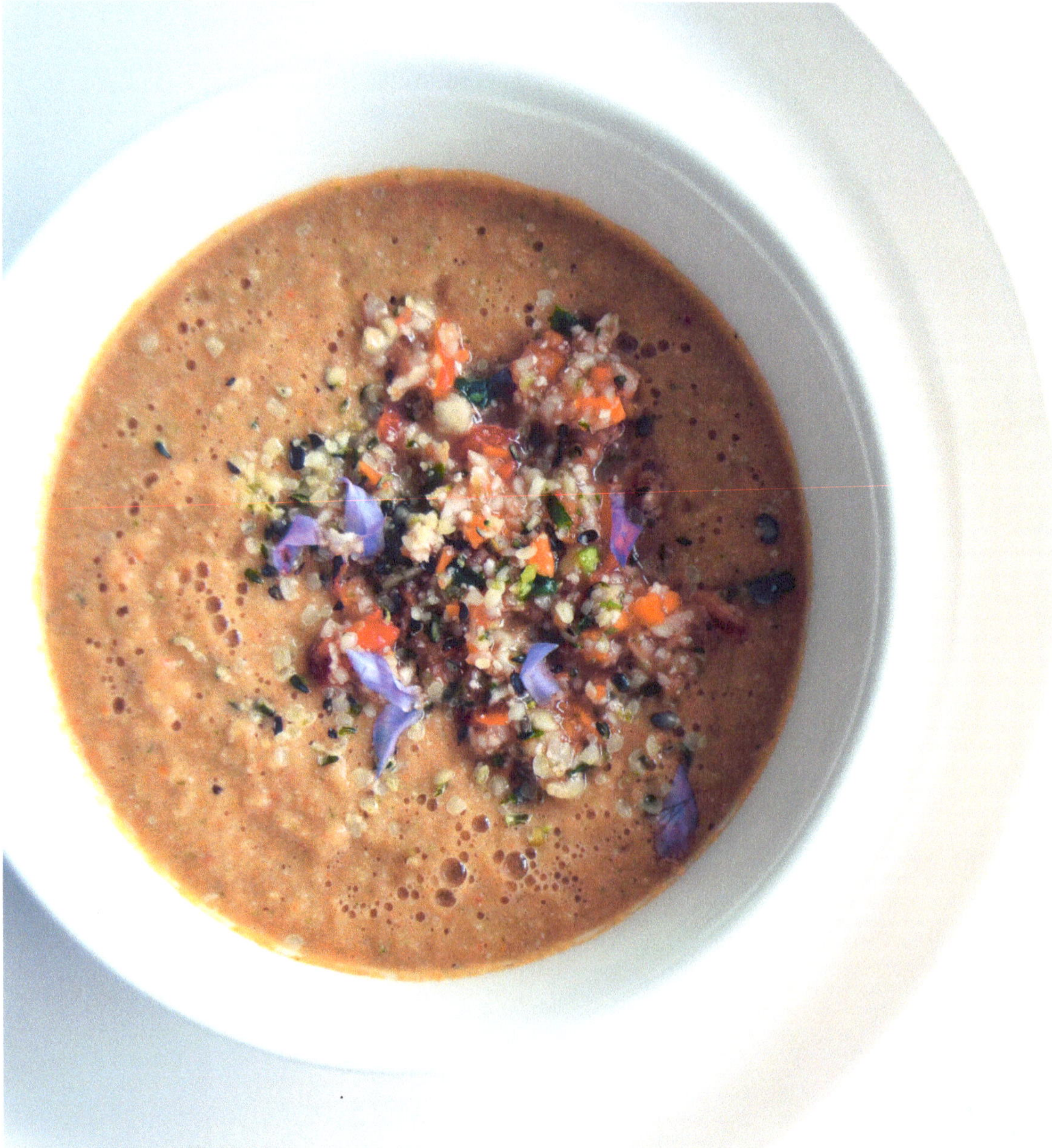

GREEK RICE SOUP

Yield: 2-4 person

Ingredients

1 small head cauliflower
1 cup green tomatoes
2 long stalks of celery
1 carrot
2 tbsp choppped onion chives
2 tbsp pumpkin seeds
1 tsp himalayan salt
2 lemon juice
1 medium red bell pepper
Borage leaves to decorate

Place the cauliflower and carrot to the food processor and process into a rice-like texture. Set aside 2 tbsp mixture for topping if you like crumby texture in your soup.

Place all remaining ingredients to the blender, mix on high speed until smooth.

Pour mixture in your bowl. Top with the remaining cauliflower carrot rice and borage leaves.

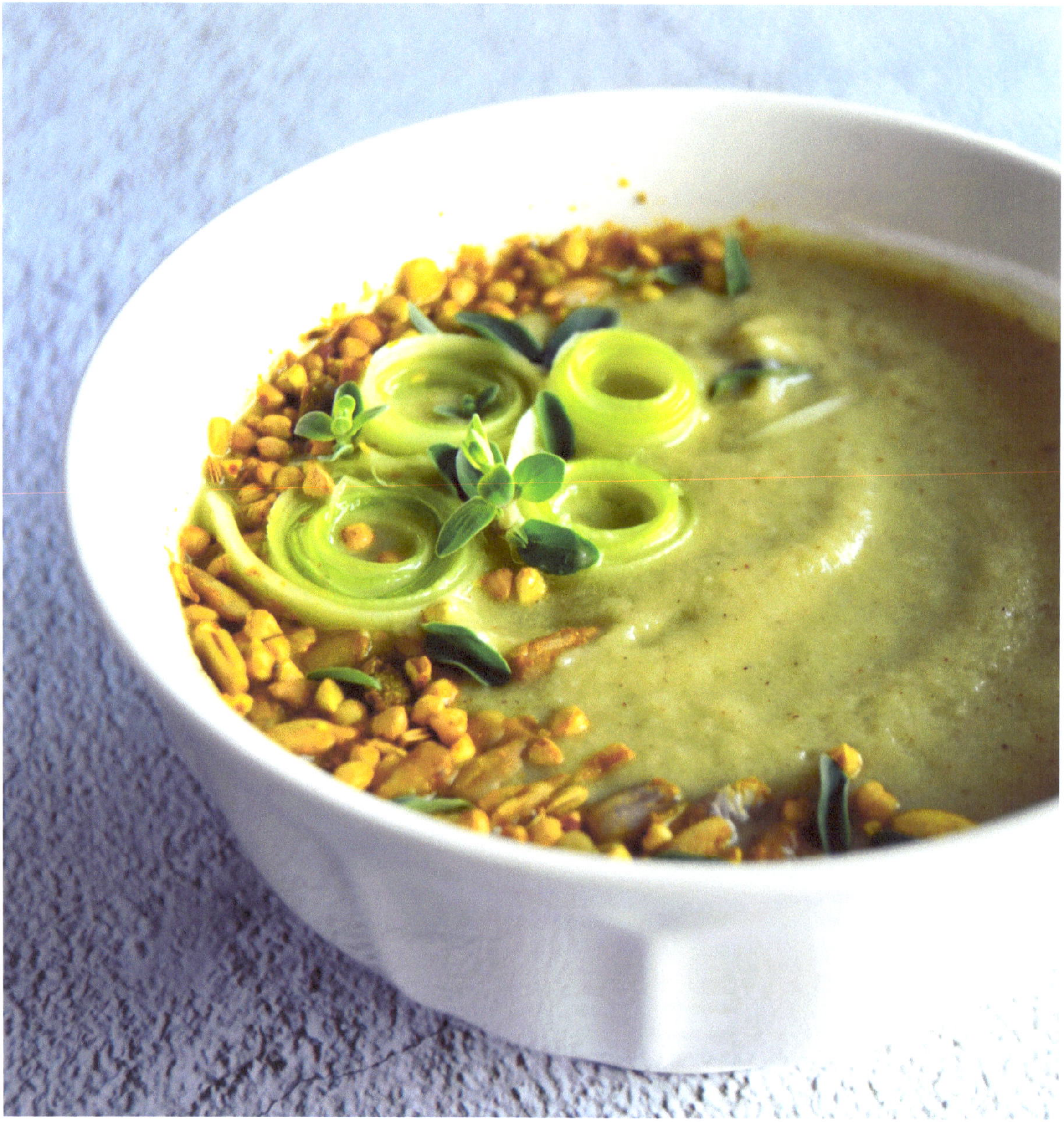

COCONUT CELERY SOUP

Yield: 2 person

Ingredients

100 ml coconut water
4 celery stalks
175 g zucchini
2 tbsp coconut butter
1/2 tsp cinnamon
A pinch pink himalayan salt

Toppings

Soaked and dehydrated sunflower seeds
Soaked and dehydrated buckwheat groats tossed with a pinch of fennel spice and cayenne
Fresh marjoram
Celery stalk trimmings rolled

Cut the zucchini into chunks. Place into blender, add all the remaining ingredients and process on high speed until you get silky smooth consistency.

Soak buckwheats and sunflower seeds, in a small bowl, mix with fennel, salt and cayenne. Dehydate until fully dried.

Using a mandoline slicer, slice celery stalk very thin. Roll into roses. Wash and drain your marjoram leaves.

Pour your soup in two small bowls. Put your celery roses on top. Sprinkle dehydrated fennel seeds, buckinis and sunflower seeds. Decorate with marjoram leaves. Drizzle a bit olive oil if desired. Serve cold or dehydrate at 42°C for 3-4 hours.

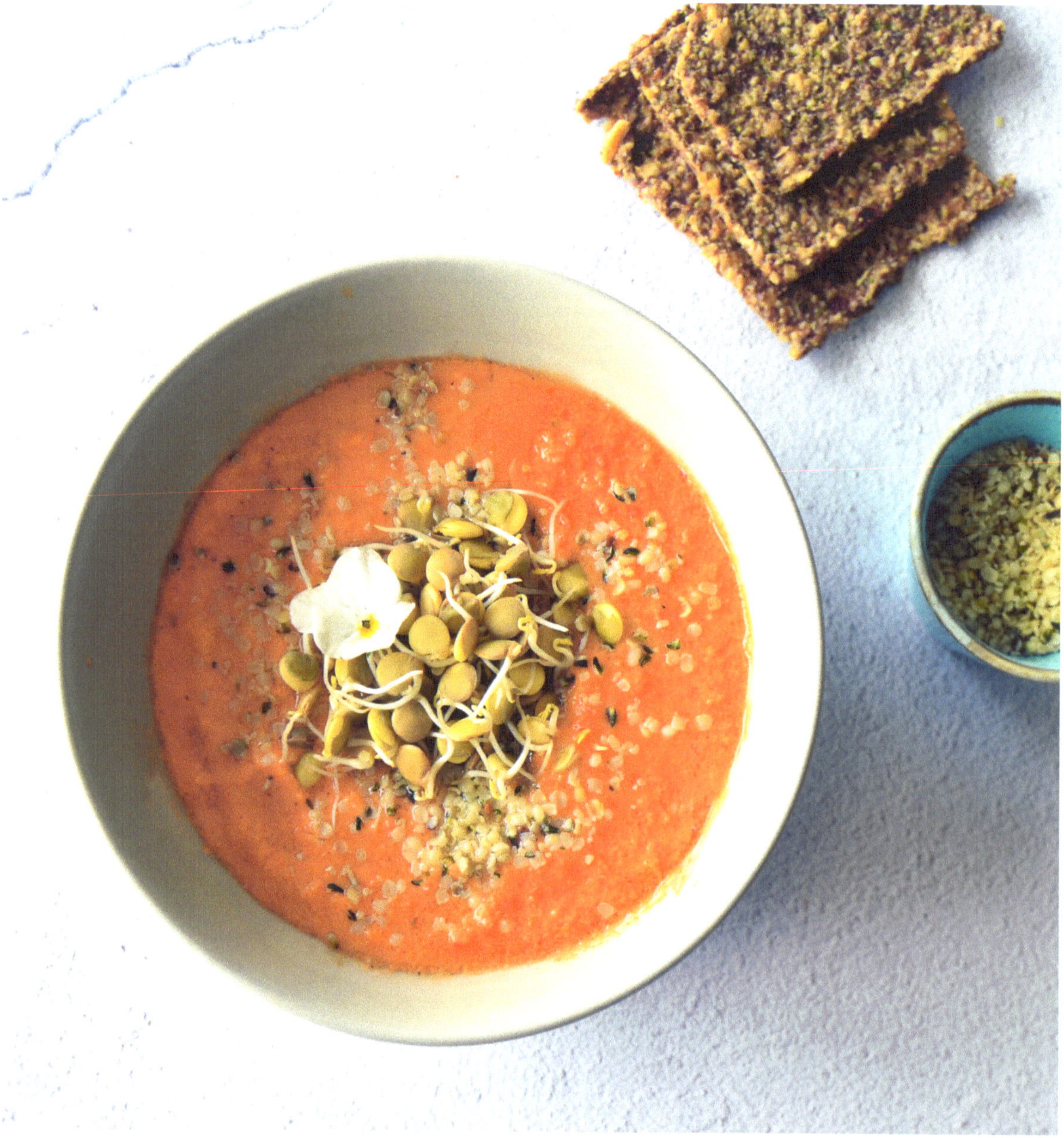

DOUBLE TOMATO SOUP WITH SPROUTED LENTILS

Yield: 2 person

Ingredients

500 g ripe tomatoes
6 pieces sundried tomatoes
7-8 brazil nuts
1 tbsp olive oil
1/4 tsp chili
1/2 tsp pink himalayan salt
250 ml filtered water
1-2 tbsp hemp hearts to serve

Sprouted Green Lentils

1 cup green lentils
2-3 lt filtered water

To sprout green lentils, place lentils in a jar and cover with water. Leave to soak overnight.
The next morning, drain and rinse your lentils. Return them to the jar without water and either cover the jar with fabric or poke holes in it's metal lid. Turn the jar upside down, propped up on chopstick for drainage and air circulation, or lay the jar on it's side. Come back to your lentils twice a day and give them a rinse and drain. After 24 hours you may start to see little tails forming. After 2 - 3 days your sprouted lentils are ready to eat.

To make the soup, place the brazil nuts in a high speed blender, mix until you get flour.
Then add the sundried tomatoes, fresh tomatoes, chili and salt. Mix until smooth.
Add the water, stir and transfer mixture in a jar or pot.
Chill until cold, about 2 hours to allow flavors to blend. Taste and season with additional salt or pepper as necessary if desired.
Divide soup between the bowls and top with sprouted lentils, hemp hearts and a drizzle of olive oil. Enjoy!

"EAT LESS, EAT RIGHT"

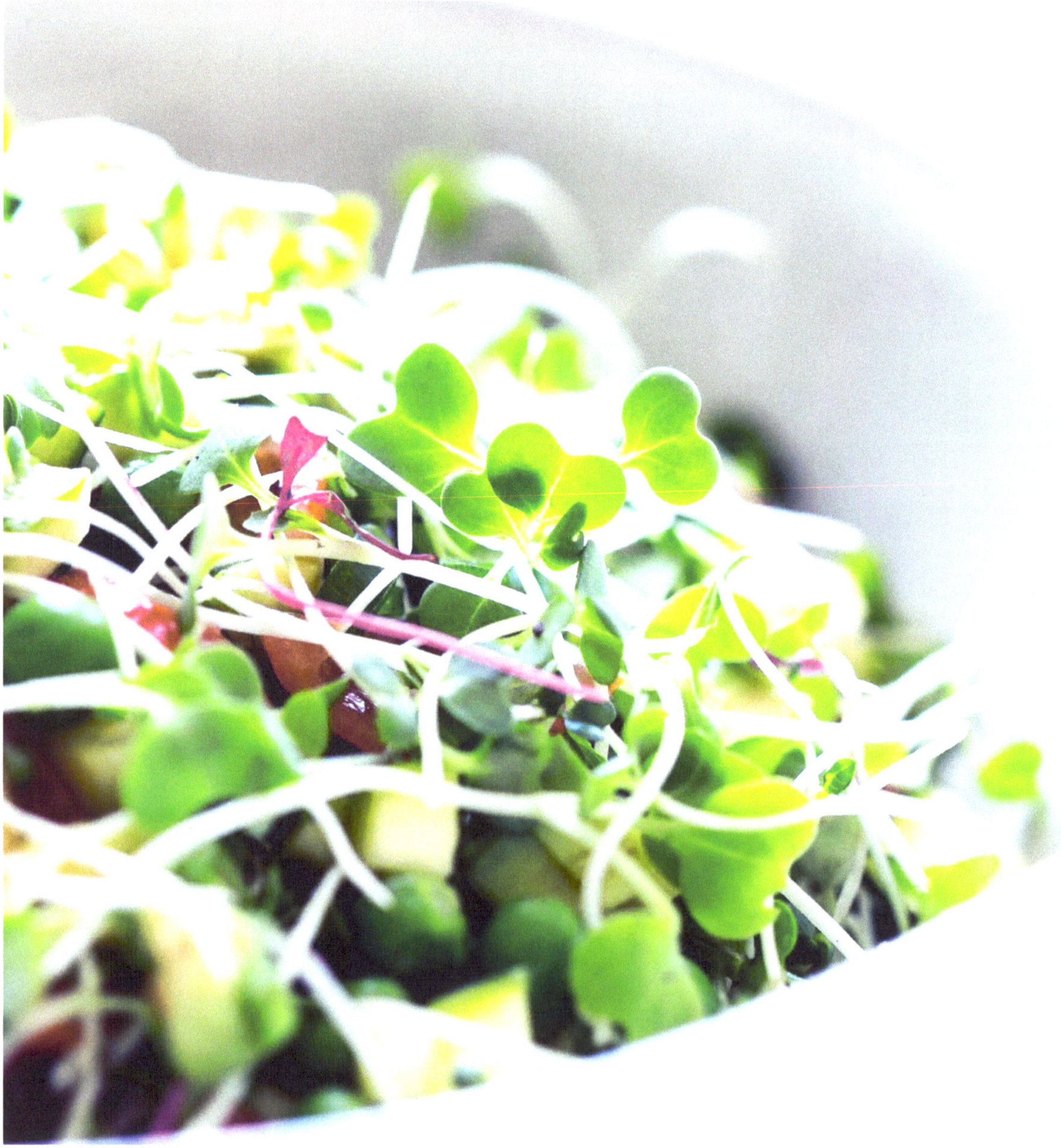

Also known as "vegetable confetti,"

SPROUTING SEEDS

WHAT IS IT?

As the name suggests, microgreens are just miniature plants of greens, herbs, or other vegetables. Like sprouts, they are a concentrated nutrient source and packed with beneficial enzymes because of their rapid growth.

Though they are often seen in dishes at gourmet restaurants because of their delicate flavor and sophisticated presentation, they are simple to grow on your own and cost very little once you have the supplies. With the right tools, you can have a year-round vegetable source on your kitchen counter

WHICH SEEDS WORK BEST?

Though Any edible plant that is entirely edible (root to leaves) can technically used, but the ones above are the most common and taste the best. Microgreens add beautiful color and great flavor to salads and are an excellent garnish for meats and other dishes.

The most common plants used for growing microgreens are:

Lettuce
Kale
Spinach
Radish
Beet
Watercress
Herbs
Greens
Cabbage
Mustard
Chia
Sunflower
Buckwheat

WHERE DO I BEGIN?

Start with a warm, sunny windowsill (direct sunlight from a south-facing window is ideal) and a small, clean container. Pie plates work well, as do clear fruit or salad boxes. If your chosen container doesn't have built-in drainage, poke a few drainage holes in the bottom. Then, prepare to plant. Read the seed packet to see if there are any special instructions.

METHOD

Cover the bottom of the container with an inch or two of moistened potting soil or mix. Flatten and level it with your hand or a small piece of cardboard, taking care not to over-compress the soil.

Scatter seeds evenly on top of the soil. Press gently into the soil using your hand or the cardboard.

Cover the seeds with a thin layer of soil. Dampen the surface with a mister. If you prefer, you can skip this step and instead cover the container with a clear lid or plastic wrap until the seeds are sprouted.

While waiting for sprouts to appear, usually within three to seven days, use the mister once or twice daily to keep the soil moist but not wet.

Once seeds have sprouted, remove the cover (if you've used one) and continue to mist once or twice a day.

Microgreens need about four hours daily of direct sunlight to thrive. In winter months, some may need even more. Leggy, pale greens are a sign of not enough sunlight. Light needs can also be satisfied with a grow light.

WHEN DO I HARVEST?

Depending upon the type of seeds you've selected, your microgreens will be ready to harvest about two to three weeks after planting. Look for the first set of "true leaves" as a sign of readiness. Then grab your scissors and snip the greens just above the soil line.

To serve, wash the microgreens with water and dry with paper towels or a salad spinner. Harvest and serve them immediately for the freshest flavor, and add to soups, salads, sandwiches or main dishes. Store remaining cut microgreens in a cotton bag in your refrigerator.

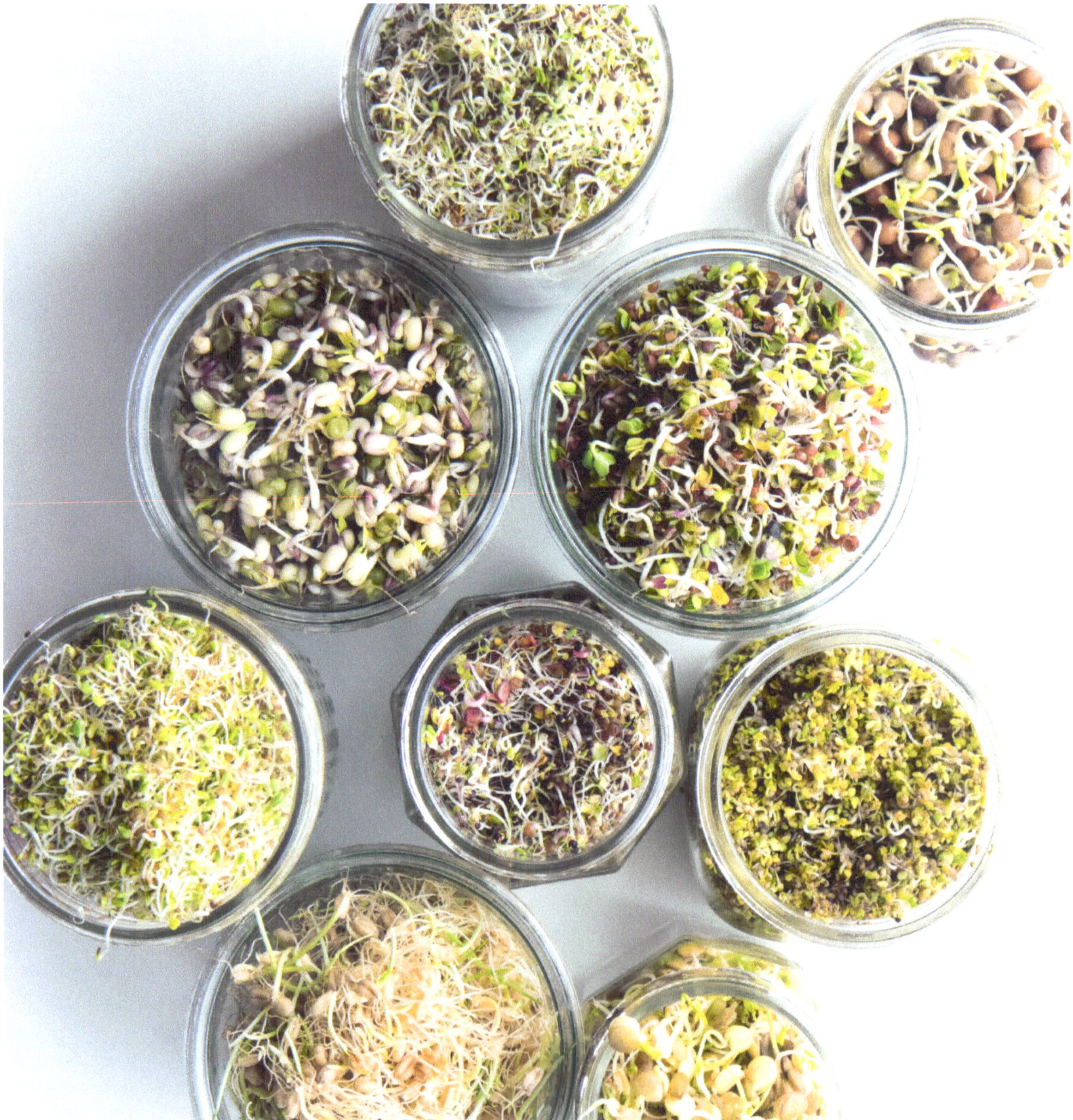

WHY JUST NOT EAT BROCCOLI?

Cruciferous vegetables have many benefits and studies find that eating them a few times a week reduces cancer risk by 30% or more. But when it comes to sulforaphane, full-grown broccoli doesn't even come close to these power-packed sprouts. In fact, 3-4 day old broccoli sprouts have up to 100x the amount of sulforaphane as mature broccoli.

On top of that, cooking destroys sulforaphane so unless you want to chow down on several pounds of raw broccoli a day, you likely won't get much (if any) sulforaphane.

BROCCOLI SPROUTS

Place two tablespoons of broccoli seeds in a wide-mouth mason jar and cover with a few inches of filtered water. Put on a sprouting lid and place the jar in a slightly warm, dark place for 8-12 hours so they can begin to sprout. The next morning (or at least 8 hours later), drain off the water and rinse with fresh water.

Rest the mason jar upside down at an angle on a sprouting jar holder or inside a bowl so that any remaining water can drain. Continue to keep the jar in a slightly warm but mostly dark place during this time.

Rinse the sprouts 2-3 times a day and place back on the jar holder or bowl after each rinse. After a few days, all of the seeds should start to break open and grow.

Keep up with the rinsing and keep the seeds in a darkish place until they have sprouts about an inch long. At this point, they can tolerate some indirect sunlight or low light exposure.

Eat the seeds once you see some dark green leaves (usually 3-4 days after the seed starts to sprout). This whole process usually takes about a week. I start a new batch every 1-2 days so we have a constant supply.

To store the sprouts:

Wait at least 12 hours from the last rinse so all remaining moisture can drain off. Replace the sprouting lid with a regular mason jar lid or transfer to an airtight container. Place in the refrigerator and store for up to a few weeks (though I recommend using them as quickly as possible).

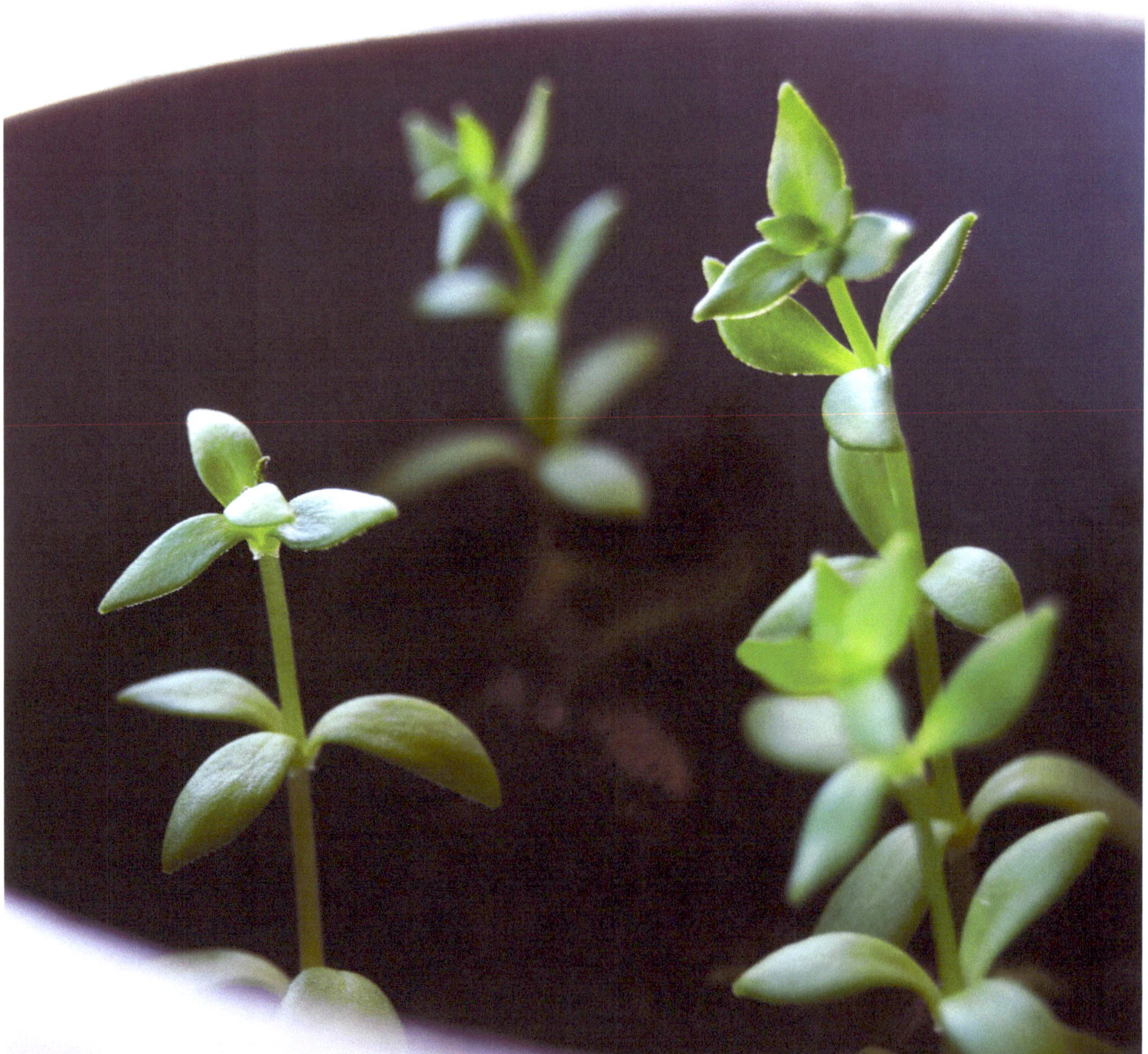

WAKE YOUR SEEDS UP

Soaking: Turning a dormant seed into a nutritional powerhouse.

Rinsing: Water is the key ingredient in sprouts. Use it liberally.

Draining: It is essential that sprouts be drained thoroughly after rinsing. Sitting in a puddle is the most common cause of crop failure.

Air Circulation: If your sprouts can't breathe while growing - they can die. Don't put them in a closed cabinet.

Greening: Photosynthesis is cool, and so is Chlorophyll, but not all sprouts are into it, nor is it necessary. Sprouts of all colors are packed with flavor and nutrition!

Cleanliness: Your seed should be clean and your sprouting device should be sterile. Wash your sprouter well between crops. Sterilize when necessary.

Storage: Properly stored, fresh sprouts will keep for up to 6 weeks in your refrigerator but fresher is better. Never refrigerate wet sprouts.

SPROUTING GRAINS

Sprouts are soaked and germinated seeds, nuts or grains that are full of beneficial enzymes, vitamins and amino acids. They are also incredibly easy to grow at home on a kitchen counter with plain water and minimal equipment.

I prefer to sprout any beans or grains that I consume to make the nutrients more bioavailable and to reduce lectins and phytic acid. I also like sprouting certain seeds and nuts for adding to salads.

Sprouts are incredibly nutritious and inexpensive, and take only a few days to grow. Sprouting increases the nutrient content of seeds and legumes and makes them easier to digest. If you've never tried to grow sprouts at home, you are missing out on an easy way to have fresh food year round.

The most common seeds used to grow sprouts are:
Chickpeas
Broccoli Seeds
Red Clover Seeds
Lentils
Mung Beans
Pumpkin Seeds
Oats
Sunflower Seeds

There is equipment specifically designed for sprouting, like sprouting trays, which make sprouting easier and allow for more growth at once, but all that is really needed are:

A wide-mouth quart size or half gallon size mason jar
A Sprouting lid or a piece of cheesecloth and a rubber band
A bowl or box to help the jar stand upside-down at an angle
Organic Sprouting seeds – Make sure they are specifically labeled "sprouting seeds" and "organic"

SOAKING VS SPROUTING

Soaking is a great way to reduce the harmful compounds in some nuts, beans and seeds by soaking them in warm water with an acidic substance (like lemon juice) added for a certain amount of time.

Sprouting is an extension of soaking. An acidic medium is not usually used, and a process if followed that allows the seed to germinate and start to grow. Some foods like beans should always be soaked before consuming, but don't necessarily need to be sprouted.

Others, especially seeds and some nuts, benefit from the additional step of sprouting.

HOW TO SPROUT MUNG BEANS?

125 g organic mung beans
3-4 lt filtered water

DAY 1
Wash mung beans , then soak them in clean water for at least 12 hours until they are double in size and the sprouts begin to appear.

DAY 2
Discard the soaking water and rinse them in clean water again. I have experienced using two tools this time-a clay pot and a vegetable washing basket. Place one layer of little mung bean sprouts on the bottom of clay pot and cover the lid. For washing basket, firstly layer a wet cloth (cotton cloth will be the best) on the bottom and lay one layer of mung bean sprouts on the surface. Cover with another wet cotton cloth. Place both of them in a dark place to avoid photosynthesis otherwise they will grow green leaves.

DAY 3
You will see some fresh green leaves. Cut the root and use it in your recipes. If you need to store, place them in a bag, sealed and keep in refrigerator for up to one week.

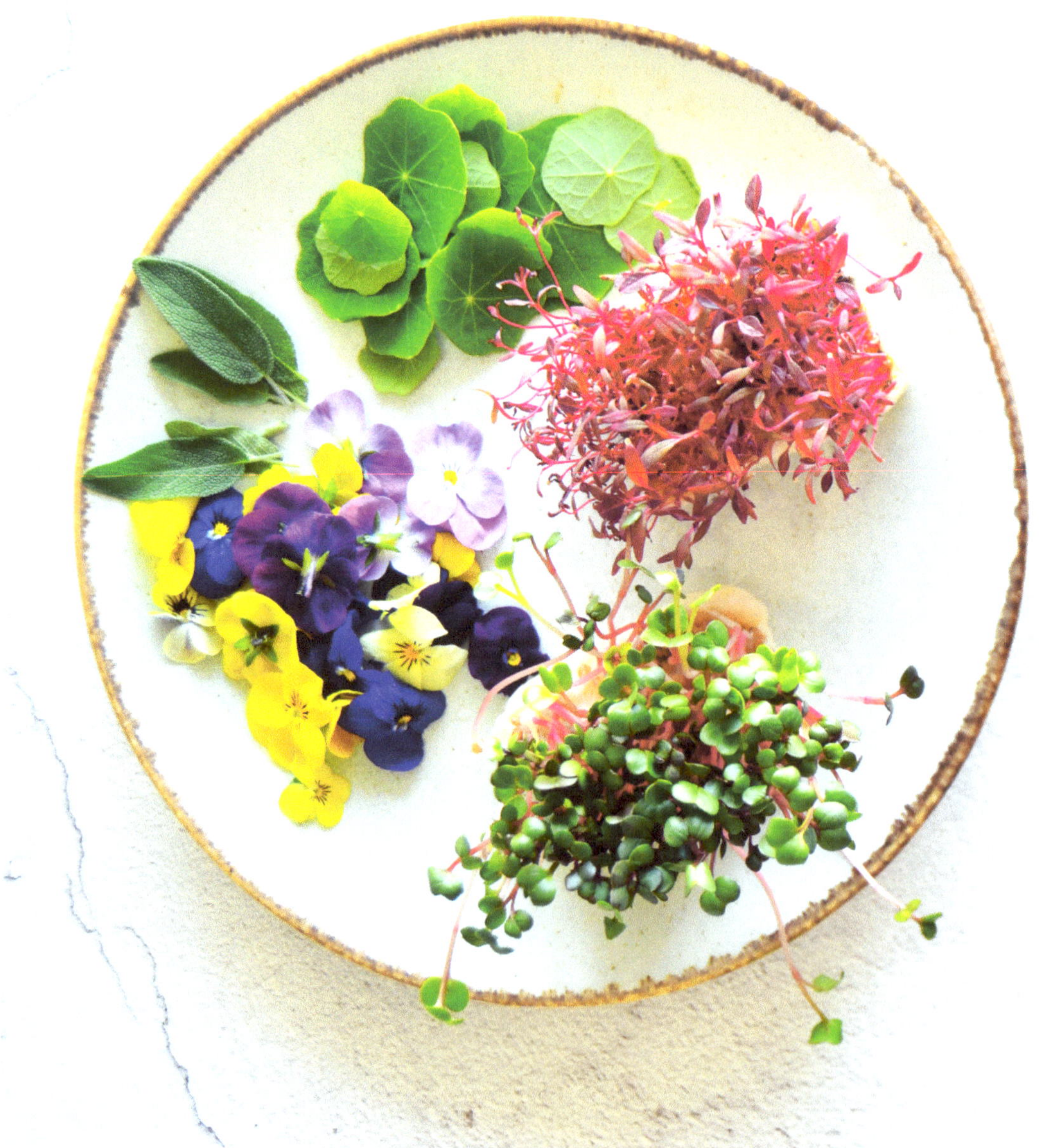

SOAKING & SPROUTING TIMES

SEED TYPE	SOAKING	SPROUTING
Almonds	8-12 Hours	No Sprouting
Pecans	4-8 Hours	No Sprouting
Macadamia	2-4 Hours	No Sprouting
Brazil nuts	3-4 Hours	No Sprouting
Cashews	4-6 Hours	No Sprouting
Tigernuts	8-12 Hours	No Sprouting
Hazelnuts	6-10 Hours	No Sprouting
Walnuts	1-2 Hours	No Sprouting
Buckwheat	6 Hours	5-7 Days
Hulled Buckwheat	20 Minutes	24 Hours
Sunflower	7 Hours	5-7 Days
Black Sesame	4 Hours	No Sprouting
White Sesame	4 Hours	No Sprouting
Flax Seeds	8 Hours	No Sprouting
Amaranth	3 Hours	24 Hours
Quinoa	4 Hours	24 Hours
Mung Beans	8-12 Hours	4 Days
Lentils	2-4 Hours	2-3 Days
Chickpeas	8 Hours	2-3 Days
Oat Groats	6 Hours	4 Days

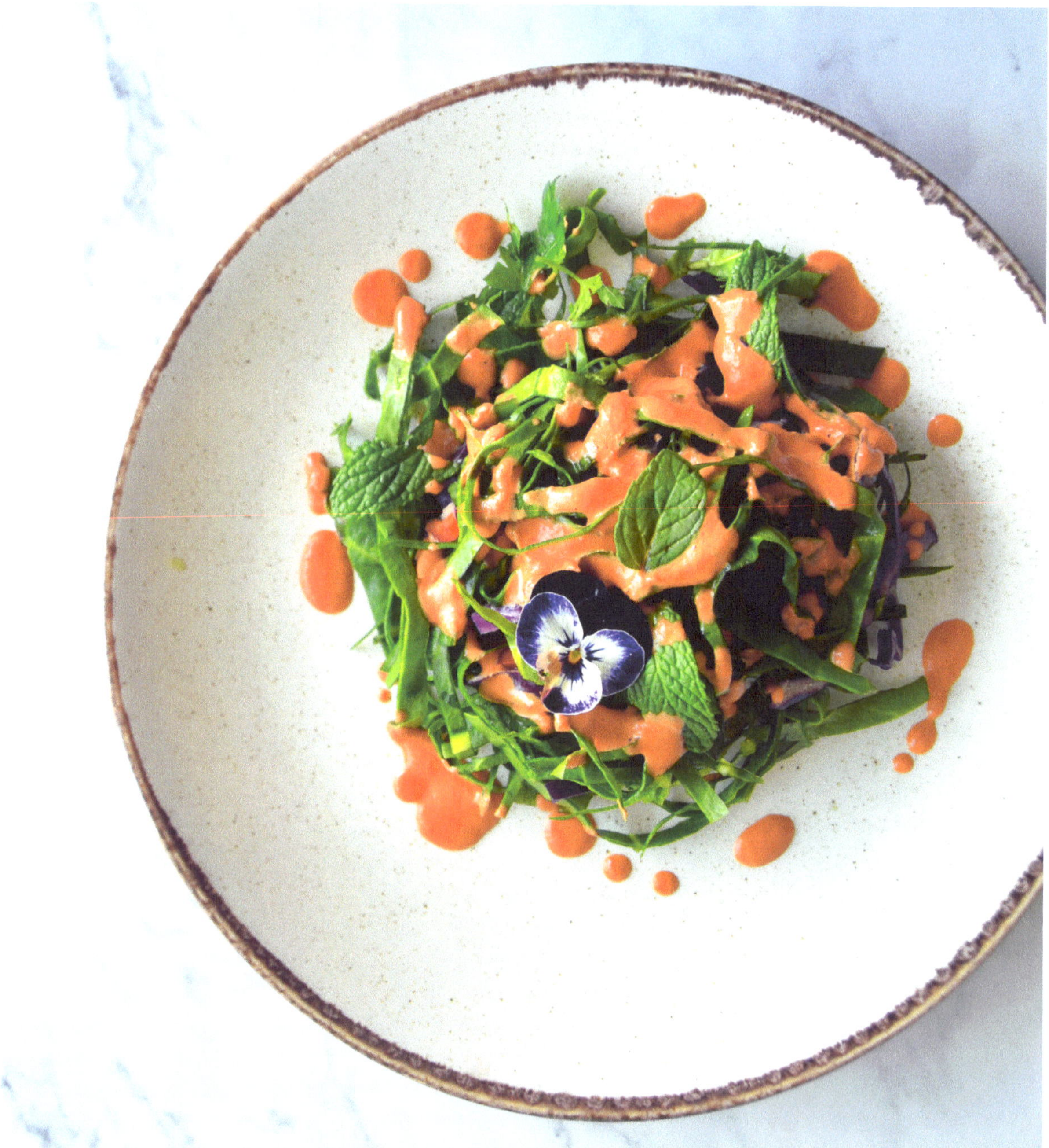

CAPSICUM SALAD DRESSING

Yield: 4

Ingredients

2 medium red bell pepper
1 large yellow capsicum
1 tbsp apple cider vinegar
2 tbsp coconut nectar
50 g sunflower seeds (or almonds, cashews, young coconut meat...)
1 tsp onion powder
1 tbsp fresh ginger grated
1/4 tsp paprika
1/2 tsp pink himalayan salt
4-5 tbsp avocado oil
1-2 tbsp lemon juice

Soak your nuts for 5-6 hours. Then strain and dry. Place in the blender, mix on high speed until you get paste. If you need add more water, one tablespoon at a time.

Add all the remaining ingredients to your blender, blend until smooth. Adjust to taste. Place in a glass bottle and pour over your favourite salad. Store in fridge for up 5-6 days.

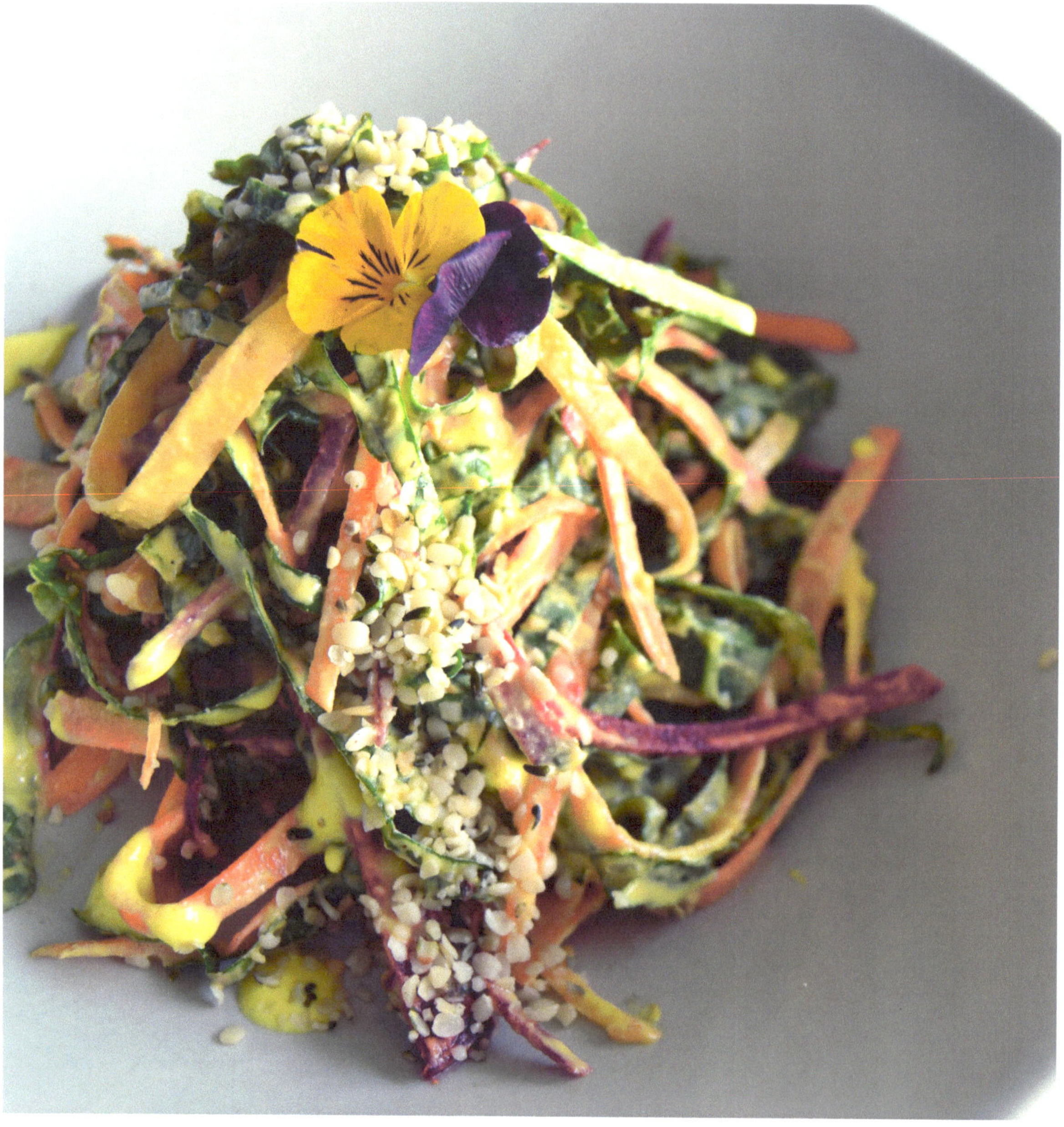

SYNCHRONIZED SALAD WITH TURMERIC DRESSING

Yield: 2 person

Sauce

50 g young coconut meat or cashews
50 ml filtered water
1 tbsp coconut oil
1 tsp apple cider vinegar
1/2 tsp turmeric
1/4 tsp pink himalayan salt
A pinch of black pepper

Salad

5-6 leaves collard greens 2-3 colorful 2-3 carrots thinly sliced
1 small beetroot spiralized

Place all the sauce ingredients in a high speed blender. Mix until silky smooth. Pour in a glass. Set aside.

Finely chiffonade the collard greens into ribbons using a sharp knife . Cut beets and carrots julienne.

Then toss with turmeric dressing in a large bowl, massaging firmly until the leaves soften.

Top with hemp hearts.

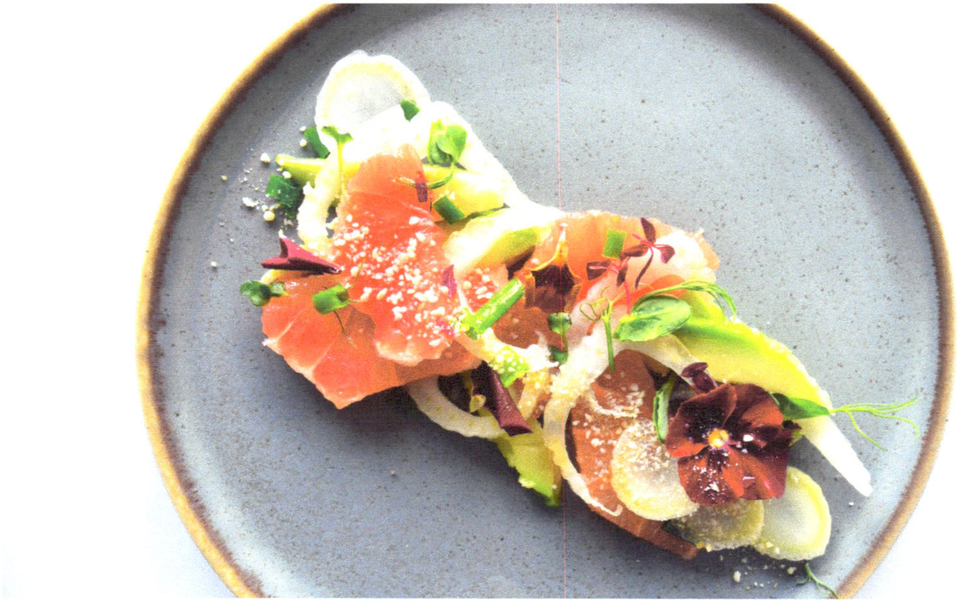

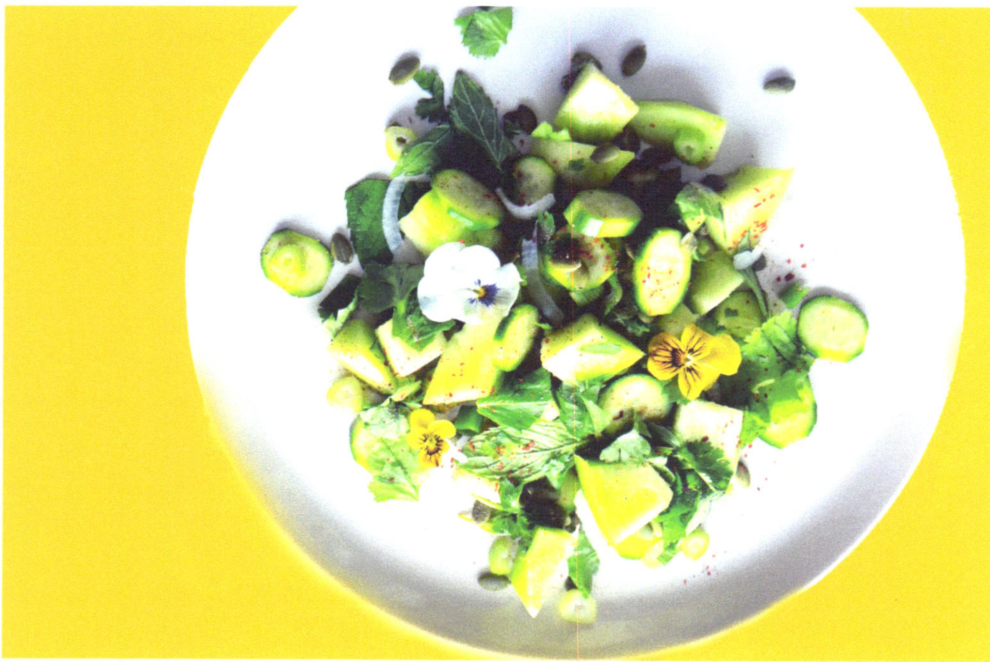

CANTALOUPE CUCUMBER SALAD

Yield: 2 person

1 cup cantaloupe cubed
1 large cucumber cubed
2 tbsp fresh mint chopped
2 tbsp chives chopped
1 tbsp cilantro chopped
1/2 tsp cardamom
A pinch of salt
1/4 tsp cayenne
2 tbsp pepitas
2 tbsp fennel stalks chopped
1/4 cup daikon shaved

Cut your cantaloupe into small chunks, slice the cucumber thinly.
Using a mandolin cutter shave daikon radish very thinly.
Cut fennel stalks thinly.

Place the cantaloupe, daikon and fennel to your plate.
Add the pepitas, chopped cilantro and mint leaves.
Sprinkle cayenne, salt and cardamom. Add hemp hearts if desired. Serve cold!

GRAPEFRUIT FENNEL SALAD

Yield: 2 person

2 pink grapefruit peeled
2 avocados peeled
1 fennel bulb thinly sliced
Rawmesan to serve
Sprouted amaranth, peas, broccoli & viola

Dressing
2 tbsp lemon juice
1 tbsp extra virgin olive oil
2 tbsp minced shallot
1 tbsp balsamic vinegar
Salt and pepper to taste

Combine the fennel, avocado, grapefruits and greens in a large bowl or plate.
Add all of the dressing ingredients into a bowl, whisk well until smooth.
Drizzle with 3-4 tablespoons of the dressing and season with the salt and pepper, top with rawmesan. Enjoy!

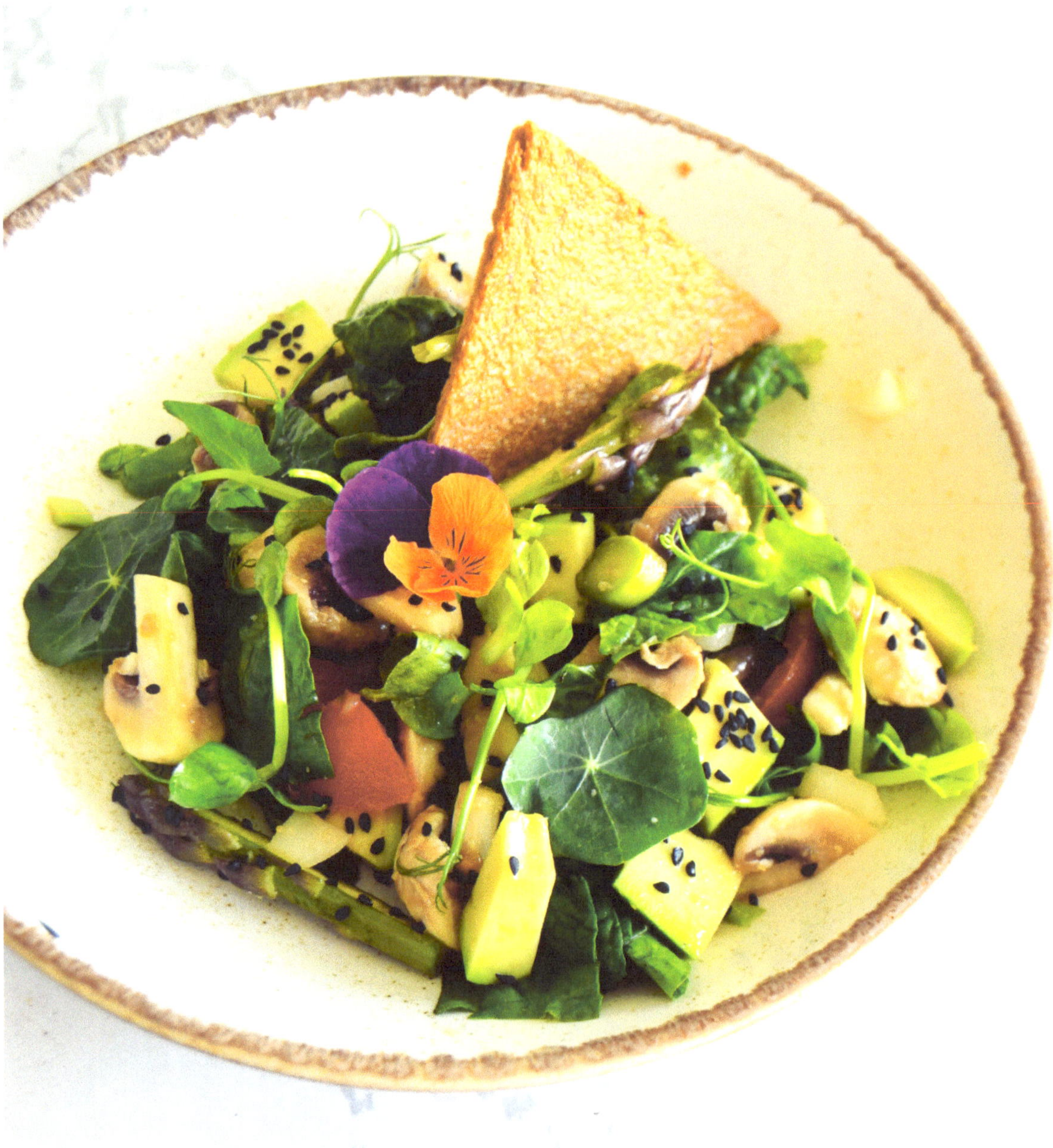

WILTED SPINACH WITH MARINATED MUSHROOMS

Yield: 2 person

Salad

2 cups spinach
1/2 lemon juice
1/2 tsp pink himalayan salt
Sesame seeds to sprinkle
Nachos bread (page 36)

Marination

1 tbsp coconut aminos
2 tbsp olive oil
1 tsp garlic powder
A pinch of cayenne
1/2 avocado
2 cups chopped mushrooms
1/2 onion thinly sliced
1 medium tomato
4 small asparagus thinly sliced

Place the spinach in a large bowl, add the lemon juice and salt. Massage with your hands and set aside. This process helps to break the spinach down and give a cooked look.

Combine all ingredients in a large bowl, toss together until mushrooms are coated well and set aside.

Add wilted spinach into the bowl and combine everything together. Let it rest at least 30 minutes. Sprinkle sesame seeds and decorate with edible flowers and pea sprouts. Then serve with nachos bread.

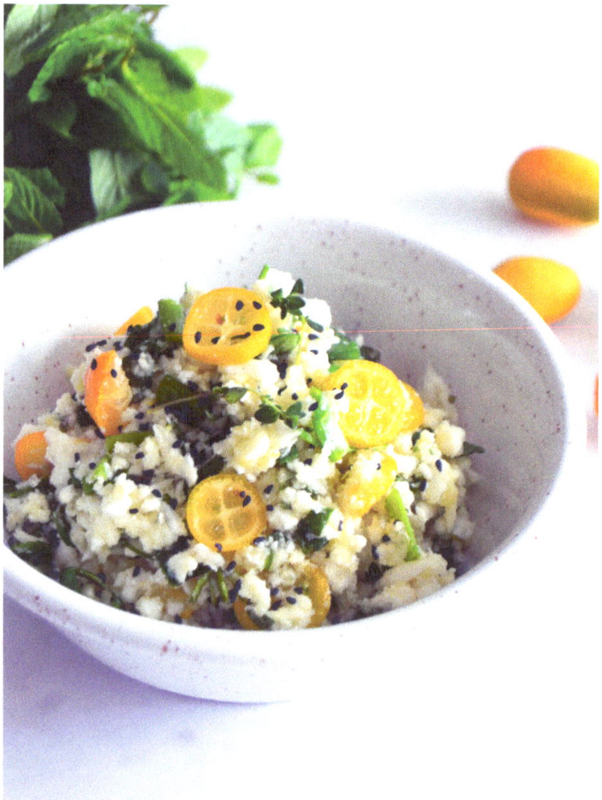

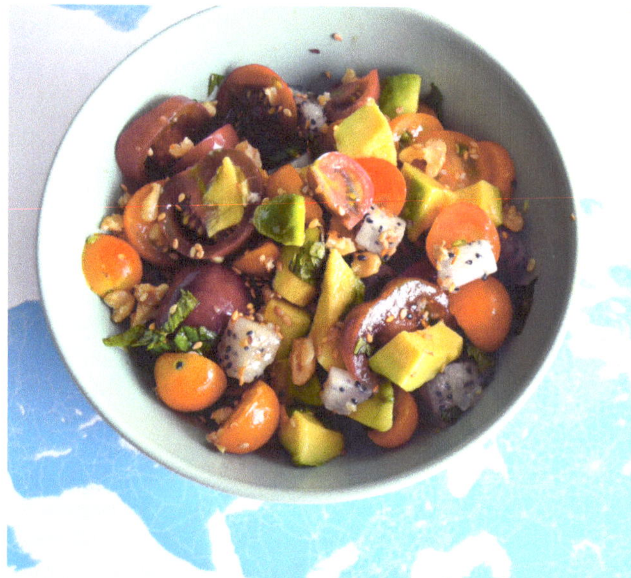

CAULIFLOWER TABBOULEH

Yield: 2 person

Ingredients

1/2 head cauliflower florets blend until rice-like texture
1 piece of lemon, grated peel and lemon juice
2 green onions, shredded
1 bunch of leaf parsley, chopped
1 bundle of mint, chopped
7-8 kumquat sliced thinly,
3 tablespoons olive oil
1 teaspoon turmeric, ground
1 teaspoon salt
1 teaspoon pepper

Tear the cauliflower coarsely and thinly slice the stem. Squeeze the excess water using a cheesecloth. Then put in a large bowl along with lemon juice and a teaspoon of salt.

Allow to marinate for about 30 minutes.

Add the remaining ingredients and mix well, taste with salt and pepper Top with kumquat slices if desired.

PITAYA AVOCADO CARPESE

Yield: 2 person

Ingredients

1 perfectly ripe pitaya diced
50 ml pomegranate juice
100 g cherry tomatoes halved
1 ripe avocado diced
1 tbsp lemon juice
1/4 cup walnut chopped
1 tsp sesame seeds
1/4 tsp salt

Wash, peel and dice your fruits. Place in a mixing bowl. Pour the lemon juice and pomegrante juice. Toss together. Then add the chopped walnuts and sesame seeds. Season with salt if needed. Enjoy!

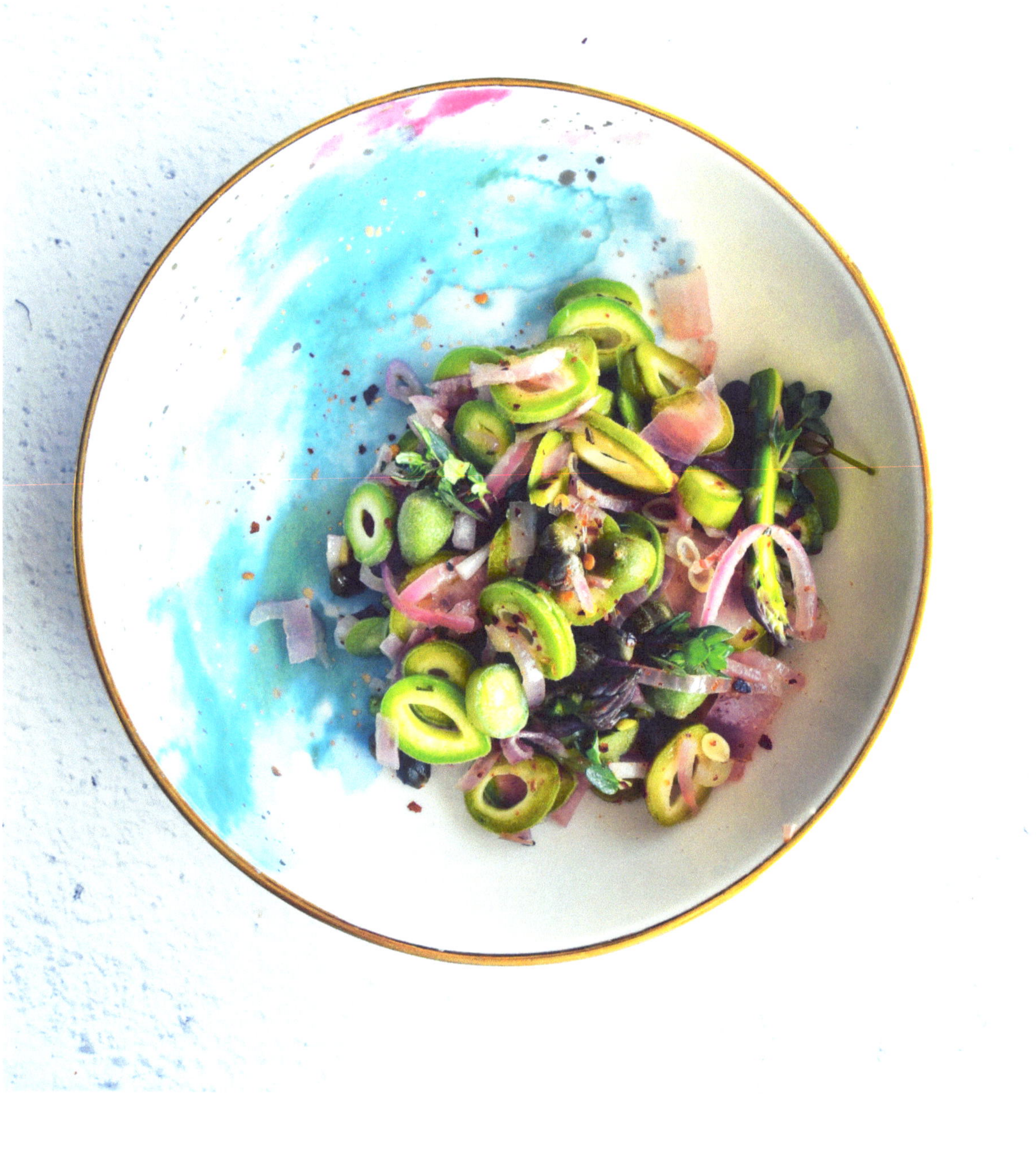

GREEN ALMOND ASPARAGUS SALSA

Yield: 2-3

Ingredients

120 g green almonds thinly sliced
1/2 bunch baby asparagus sliced thinly
1 medium red onion thinly sliced
2 tbsp red wine vinegar
2 tbsp pickled capers
A pinch of salt and chili pepper to taste
1 tbsp olive oil (optional)
1/4 bunch fresh thyme chopped
1/4 bunch fresh parsley chopped (optional)

In a mixing bowl, toss the chopped onions, asparagus, green almonds, pepper and a pinch of salt with the red wine vinegar. Set aside to macerate for at least 15 -20 minutes.

Next, add the capers, parsley and thyme to the bowl with marinated green almonds. Slowly whisk in the olive oil. Add salt and pepper to taste. Enjoy!

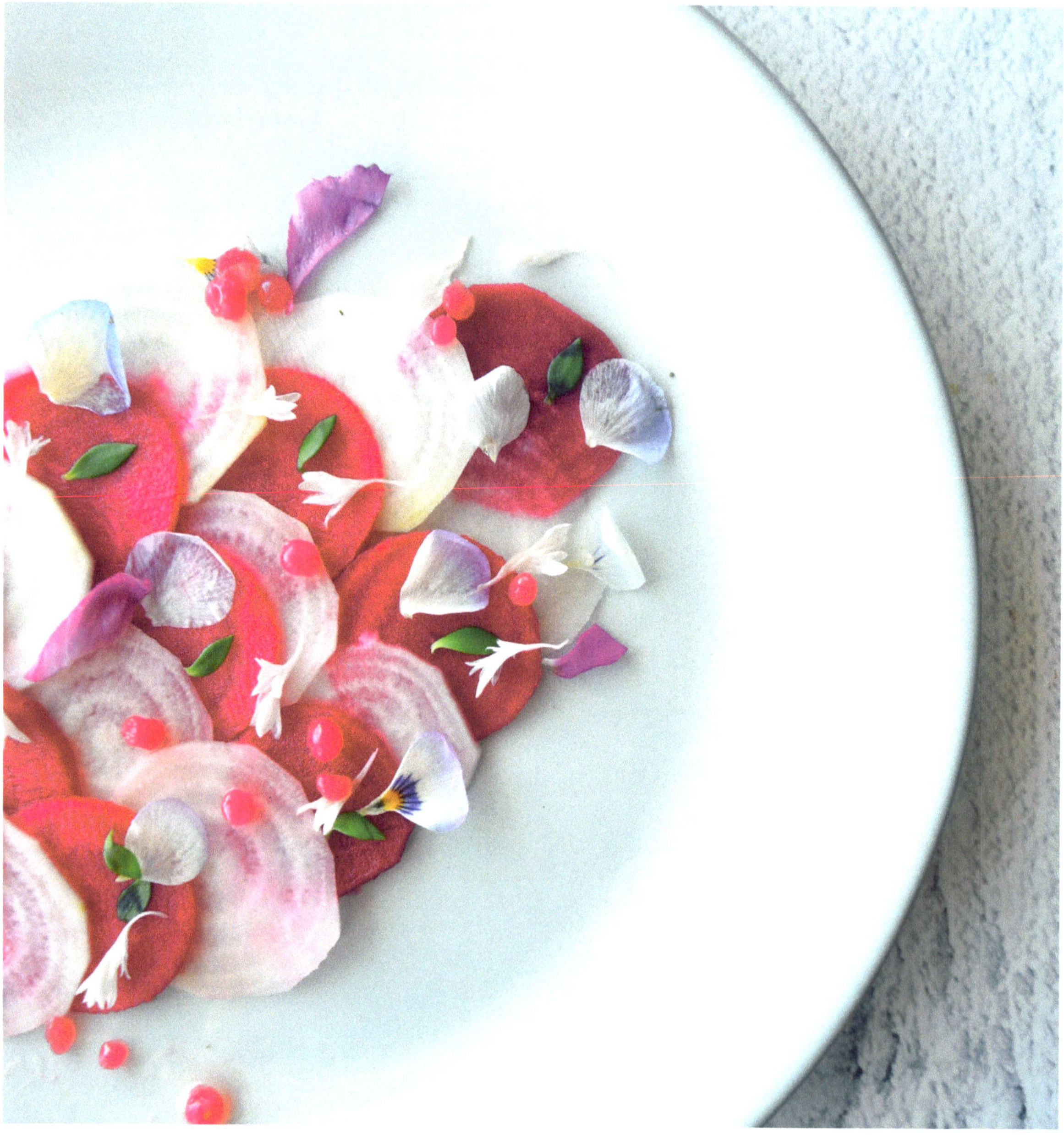

BEET CARPESE WITH STRAWBERRY PEARLS

Yield: 2 person

Ingredients
2 small white beets
2 small red beets
3 tbsp white grape vinegar

Strawberry Pearls
150 g fresh strawberry juice
1 tbsp coconut water
1 tbsp maple syrup
1/2 cup irish moss
1/4 cup water

For Garnish
White corn flower petals
Gangnam tops

Using a mandolin, slice beets very thinly.
Place white and red beets in seperate bowls in order to prevent color change.
Drizzle white grape vinegar, let it sit overnight.
Pour extra virgin olive oil into a tall glass and set in the freezer. Let stand for about 4 hours so that it gets really cold.
Mix irish moss and water well in blendec twister jar. When you get puree, add the strawberry juice.
Blend well until smooth. If it is too thick add a little bit water. We need it in liquid form in order to squeeze.
Then transfer mixture to a syringe. Squeeze small drops into the oil. They will form into small drops and slowly sink to the bottom.
Lift up the drops at regular intervals and rinse them in a sieve under cold water. Put aside.
Strain the beets in the mornging and dry using a paper. Lay them as one white and one red in a large plate.
Place some strawberry pearls on them and decorate with cornflower petals and gangnam. Enjoy!

TIPS
Alternatively you can spread 1 inch thick onto a loaf pan. Refrigerate for 4 hours. With the end of a small tea spoon, lift out a very small pearl size.

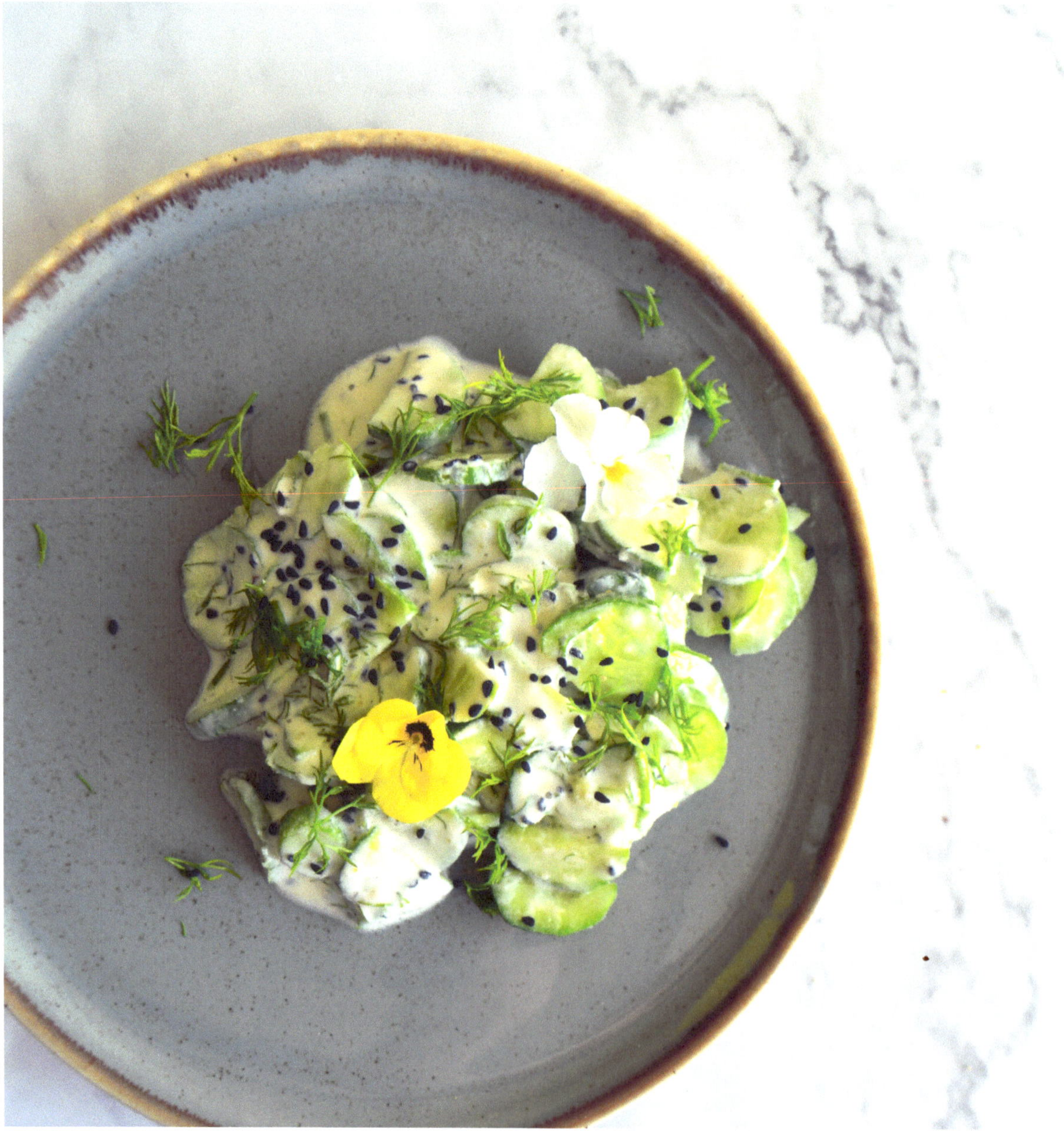

CREAMY CUCUMBER SALAD

Yield: 2 person

Ingredients

2 large english cucumber
1/2 cup cashew yogurt
1/2 bunch fresh dill chopped
1/4 tsp sea salt
Juice of 1/2 lemon
2 tbsp black sesame seeds
2 garlic cloves minced

Peel the cucumber and slice in half lengthways or using a spiral cutter make cucumber noodles.

Place cucumber to a large bowl.

Chop the dill finely , stir the lemon juice, yoghurt and minced garlic.

Pour mixture over the cucumber. Toss together. Sprinkle black sesame seeds. Serve cold!

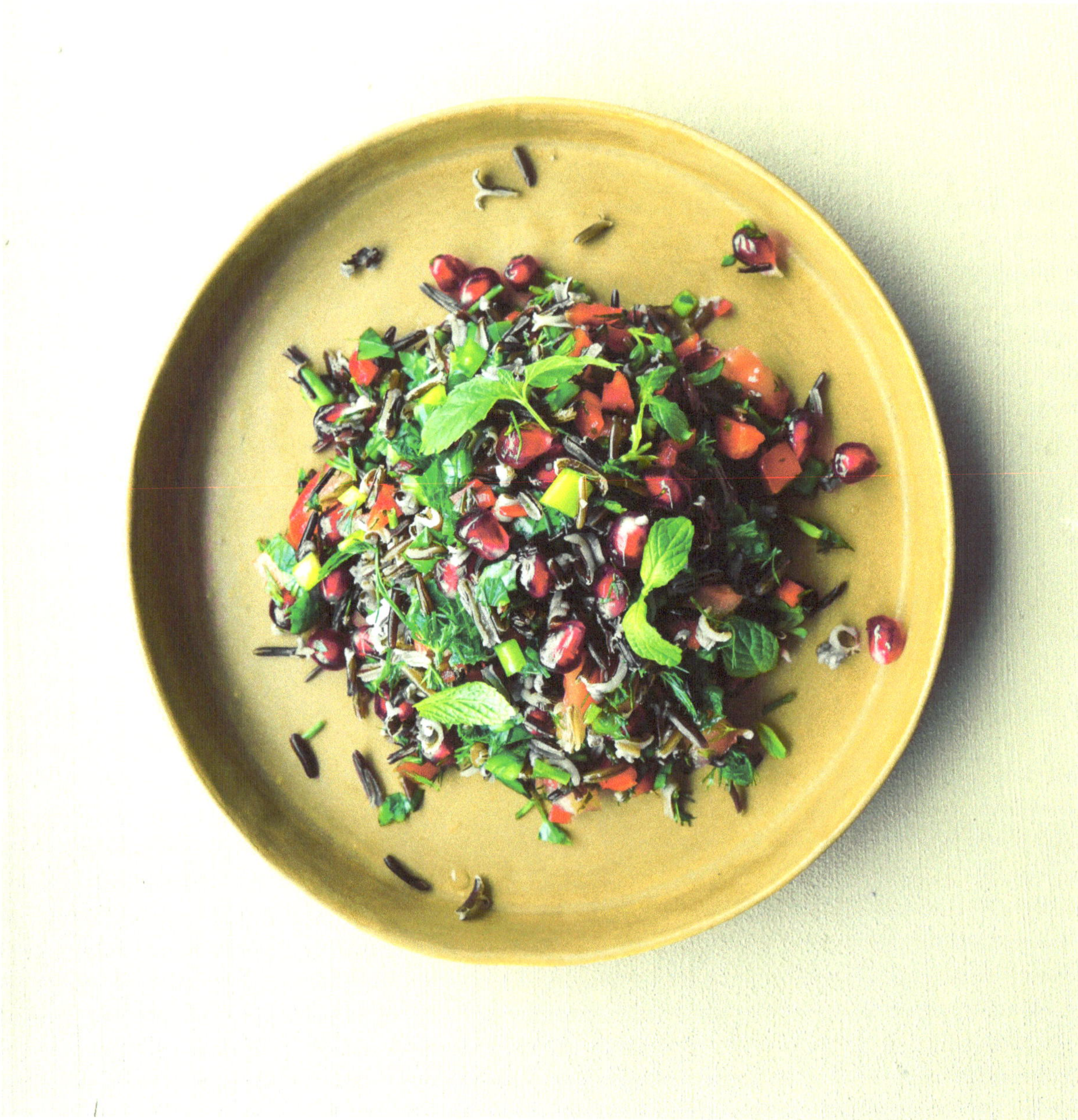

BLOOMED BLACK WILD RICE TABBOULEH

Wild black rice is not a rice or grain at all in fact, but the seed of aquatic grass that grows along the shores of fresh-water lakes in the Northern US. It is a complete protein with a full amino acid profile, also has more protein and fiber than the other rices. The glycemic index is also lower than the white and brown rice due to its higher protein and fiber content and it's rich, nutty flavour pairs well with fresh zingy flavours.

Yield: 2 person

Ingredients

90 g wild black rice (blackened or wood-parched)
1 cup pomegranate seeds
1 large tomato
1 large red bell pepper
1/4 cup fresh mint leaves
1/4 cup fresh mint leaves
1 cup fresh parsley
1/2 cup fresh dill
1/4 cup green onions
Juice of 1 whole lemon
Salt and pepper to taste

Place the wild black rice in a pot, cover with water. Let it soak at least 12-14 hours or overnight. Then rinse well. Eating any other rice raw is not recommended. Black rice blooms when soaked overnight, and this is why it can be eaten raw. The hard outer shell of the black rice (also known as the hull) will bloom during overnight soaking. Blooming means the rice softens and the hull breaks open exposing the innards of the rice as if it were cooked. So even though it's raw, it has the texture of being cooked.
Chop your herbs finely, cut the red bell pepper and tomato into small cubes.
In a large mixing bowl, mix all bloomed rice with the rest of the ingredients together. Give them a good toss.
Taste, adjust the salt and pepper.

Notes: Note: Do not confuse forbidden black rice with wild rice. Both are black in color, but they are not the same thing!

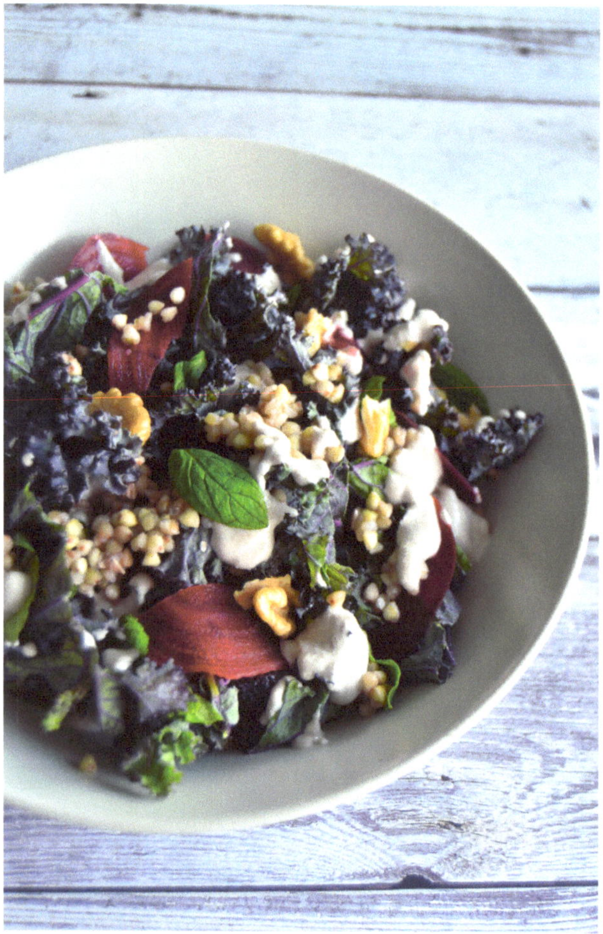

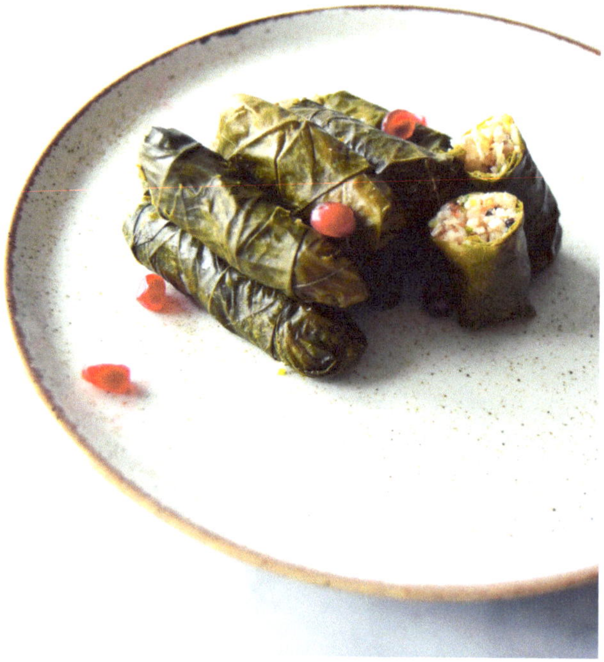

RAWMA DA VINCI - RAW DOLMAS

Yield: 4-6 person

Ingredients

2 cups grape leaves to wrap
1 medium cauliflower (700 g)
1 medium zucchini
1 cup tomato
1 tsp garlic powder
2 tbsp hemp hearts
2 tbsp sunflower seeds
2 tbsp chopped onion chives
2 tbsp lemon juice
1 tsp pink himalayan salt
2 tbsp chopped dill

Place all filling ingredients into a high speed blender, mix until finely chopped. Transfer mixture in a bowl set aside.

Place fresh grape leaves in the water, soak for 10-15 minutes. Then strain and drain. Set aside.

Place 1 tbsp of the mixture into the center of each grape leaf and roll into a small long roll. Place rolls in a dehydrator. and set to 107° F for 2 – 2.5 hours, remove and serve!

BUCKWHEAT KALE SALAD WITH WALNUT DRESSING

1 beet finely sliced
1 cup kale chopped
1/4 cup fresh mint
1/2 cup buckwheat sprouted
1/2 cup walnut chopped
1/4 cup dried figs chopped

Walnut Dressing

4 tbsp lemon juice
1 cup raw walnuts
1 tbsp hemp oil
Water to thin
Salt and pepper to taste

Place chopped kale leaves into the bowl
Thinly slice beets using a mandolin slicer.
Remove steems of the mint, wash and drain the leaves.
Place all dressing ingredients into the food processor, mix on high speed until smooth.
Pour over the kale leaves, massage well.
Add the sprouted buckwheats.
Add the chopped walnuts and figs. Serve!

ZUCCHINI SAMOSAS WITH MINT RAITA

Yield: 4-6

Samosa

2 large zucchini
2 tsp garam masala
1/2 tsp chili powder
3 tbsp olive oil
1/4 cup golden flax meal

Base

1/4 cup soaked cashews
1 ripe avocado
1 tsp garlic powder
1/4 cup chopped fresh mint
1 tbsp lemon juice
1/2 tsp pink himalayan salt

Filling

1 cup sunflower seeds
2 tbsp coconut aminos
1 tbsp lemon juice
1 tsp garlic powder
1 tsp ginger powder
1/4 tsp turmeric
5 sundried tomato halved
1/2 tsp himalayan salt
3 tbsp filtered water
a pinch freshly ground black pepper
1/4 tsp red pepper flakes
1/2 tsp onion powder
1 small zucchini peeled
1/2 cup fresh spinach

Instructions

Blend all samosa ingredients except flax meal in a high-speed blender until well combined.

Add flax meal and blend again until smooth.

Pour mixture onto a nonstick dehydrator sheet and spread evenly into a square. (26x26 cm)

Dehydrate for 8 hours at 46°C , or until able to peel off the sheet. Once the nonstick sheets are removed, return to the dehydrator for 30 minutes, until both sides are dry to the touch but still pliable.

To make filling, place all ingredients into the food processor, chop until crumble and combined well.

To make mint raita, place all mint raita ingredients into the food processor mix on high speed until you get fluffy texture.

To assemble, cut the wrappers into strips approximately 7 cm by 25 cm, and fold over the corner of one end. Fill with the mixture. Fold the pointed end. Tuck the corner in so it doesn't stick out. Start folding the remaining part of the wrapper around so it forms that familiar triangle shape.

CUCUMBER AVOCADO ROLLS

Yield: 2

For the Rolls

2 large english cucumber,
2 tbsp black sesame
1/2 cup sprouted peas

For the Cream

1 ripe avocado,
1/2 tsp pink himalayan salt,
2 tbsp fresh lemon juice,
1 tsp onion powder,
1 tsp garlic powder
3-4 slices of fresh jalapeno

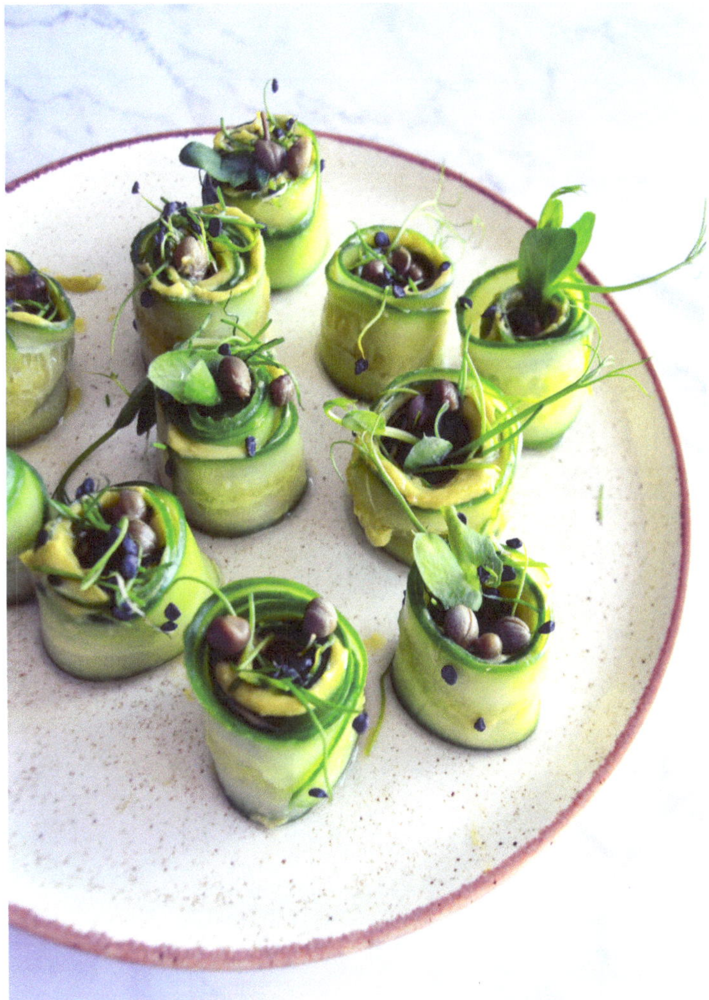

Instructions

Wash and dry your cucumbers. Use a mandolin to cut thin slices all the way through. Keep slicing the sides until you reach the full centre. Place all sauce ingredients in the food processor, mix on high speed until you get silky smooth mixture. Lay out each cucumber slice and layer a coat of the avocado spread all the way across. Start to roll on one side until you reach the end. Dress up with sprouted pea and sesame. Serve!

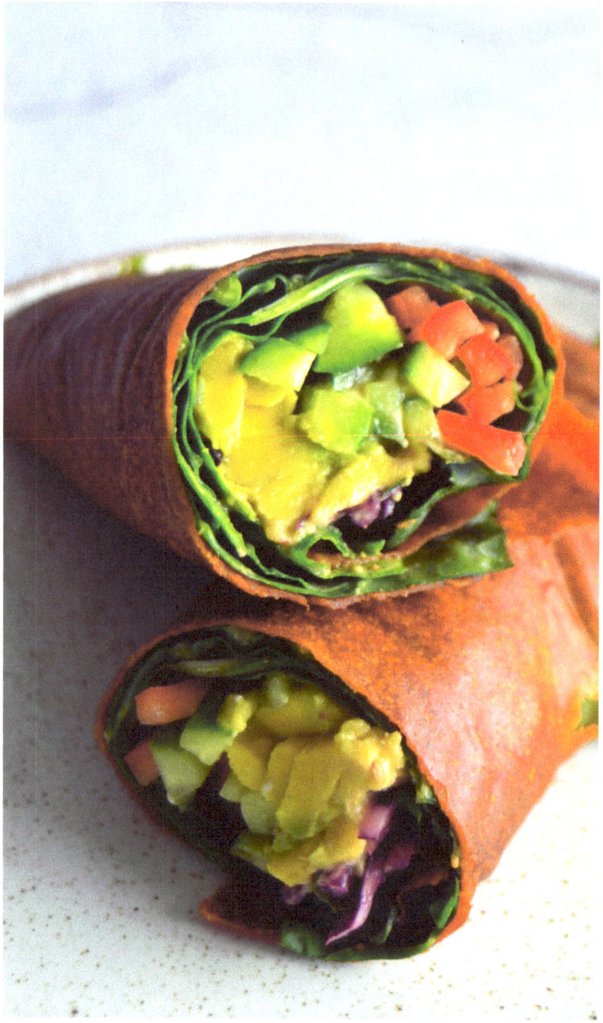

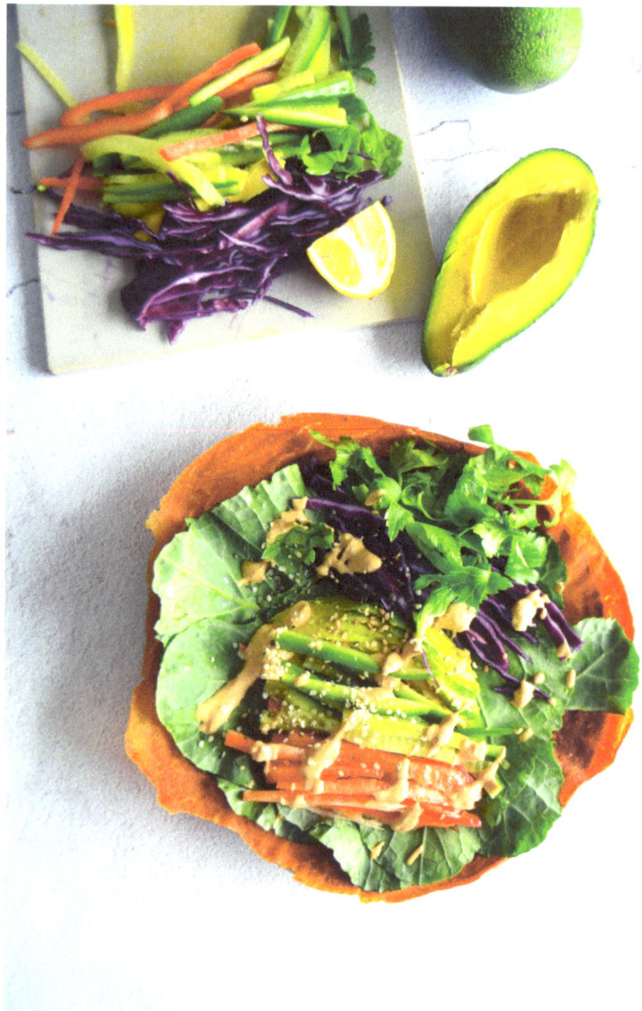

HARISSA CARROT WRAPS

Yield: 2 person

Wrap
50 g flaxseed meal,
220 ml. filtered water,
270 g carrot pulp,
80 g red bell pepper chopped,
40 g cherry tomatoes chopped,
1 tbsp lemon juice,
1/2 tsp harissa spice,
1/4 tsp cayenne,
1 tsp salt

Filling
Thinly sliced purple cabbage, green collards, cucumber, avocado, parsley, red bell pepper and cultured cashew cream or vegan tzatziki sauce or guacamole.

Blend all the wrap ingredients in a blender or food processor until very smooth. The consistency should be fluid. 2. Spread mixture onto the parchment sheets approximately 4 mm (3/16 inch) thick using a angled spatula.
Dehydrate at 41°C (106°F) for 7-8 hours, or until the exposed side has set and is firm enough for you to peel away from the sheets.
Flip the wrap onto a mesh tray and peel back the sheets. If you need, dehydrate for a further 1-2 hours or until completely dry but still pliable. (You should be careful and do not to over-dry the wraps. If the wraps become too dry and start cracking around the edges)
Once ready, cut each sheet into 2-4 pieces using a sharp knife, depending on how large you like your wrap. Store them in single layers in an air-tight container with parchment paper between each layer to prevent sticking in the refrigerator up to 2-3 weeks.
To roll them, place 4-5 green collard leaves on the carrot wraps. Slice veggies very thinly according to your preference, place on the collard leaves, spread cashew cream or guacamole sauce, sprinkle sesame seeds and roll it carefully. Enjoy!

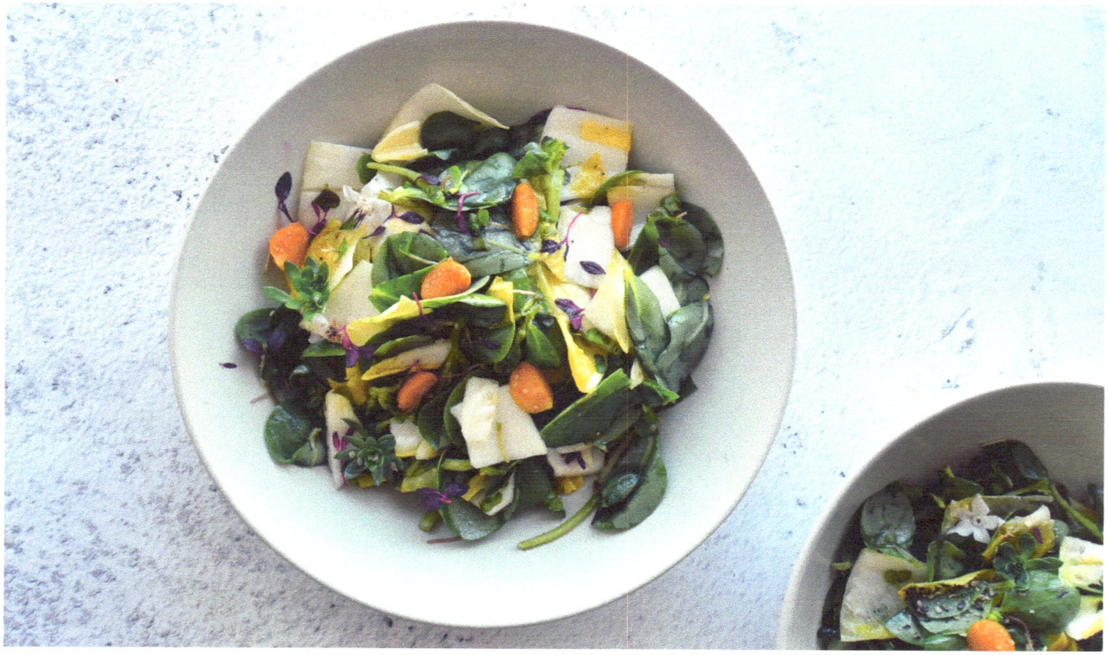

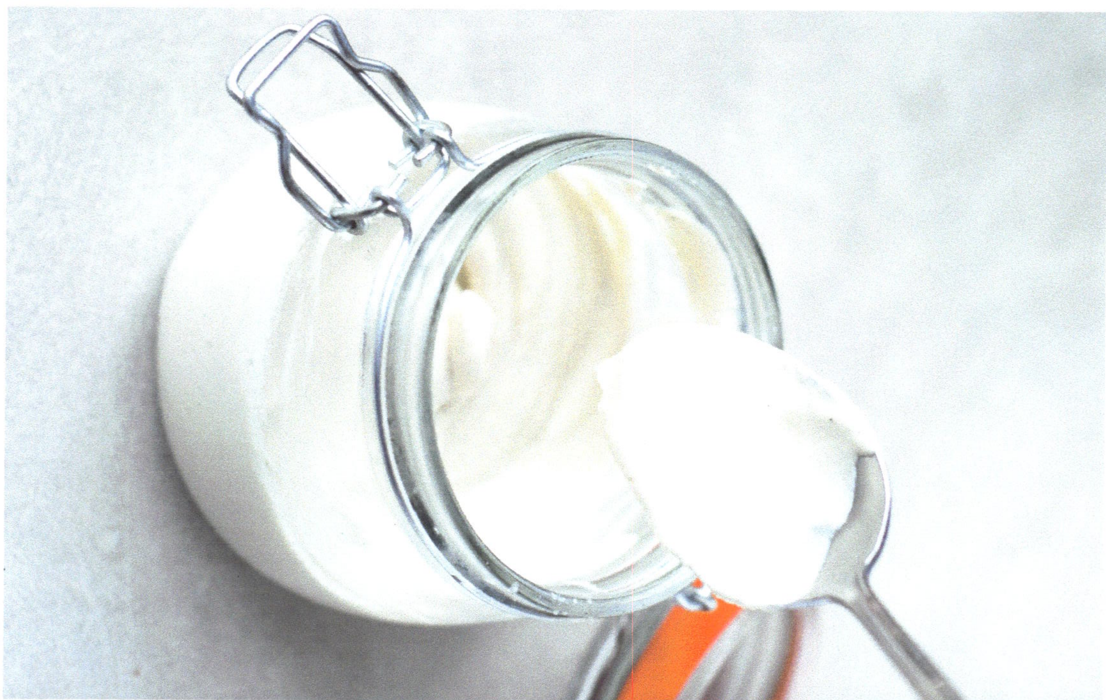

ENDIVE WILD PURSLANE SALAD

Yield: 2

Ingredients

2 heads endive chopped
4 cups purslane
1 cup radish microgreens
1/2 cup microgreens of your choice
4-5 fresh physalis halved
Hemp hearts for topping

Dressing

1 tbsp apple cider vinegar
1 tsp dijon mustard
2 tbsp extra virgin olive oil
Salt and pepper to taste

To prepare endive for salads, first remove the crunchy core: Using a paring knife, halve the endive lengthwise and make two angled cuts along the outside of the core. Pull out and discard the core, and then slice. Place in a large bowl.
Wash your purslane, gangam tops and microgreens. Transfer to the bowl.
Add vinaigrette ingredients into a small bowl. Whisk well until well combined.
Toss with greens and top with hemp hearts and halved physalis. This salad also can be served sour cashew yogurt (recipe is given below)

SOUR CASHEW YOGURT

Yield: 4

Ingredients

200 g raw cashews
2 probiotic capsules
130 ml filtered water
1/4 tsp sea salt
3 tbsp lemon juice
1/4 tsp mint (optional)

Soak the cashews overnight. Strain and place in a high speed blender. Add water and probiotic capsules. Mix on high speed until you get silky smooth mixture.

Transfer mixture in a bowl, cover with a kitchen towel. Dehydrate for 8-10 hours at 30 ° C

After fermentation process , add salt, mint and lemon juice. If the mixture is too intense, add 2-3 tbsp water and stir well. Transfer in a mason jar. Chill and use in your recipes.

Store in the refrigerator for up to 4-5 days.

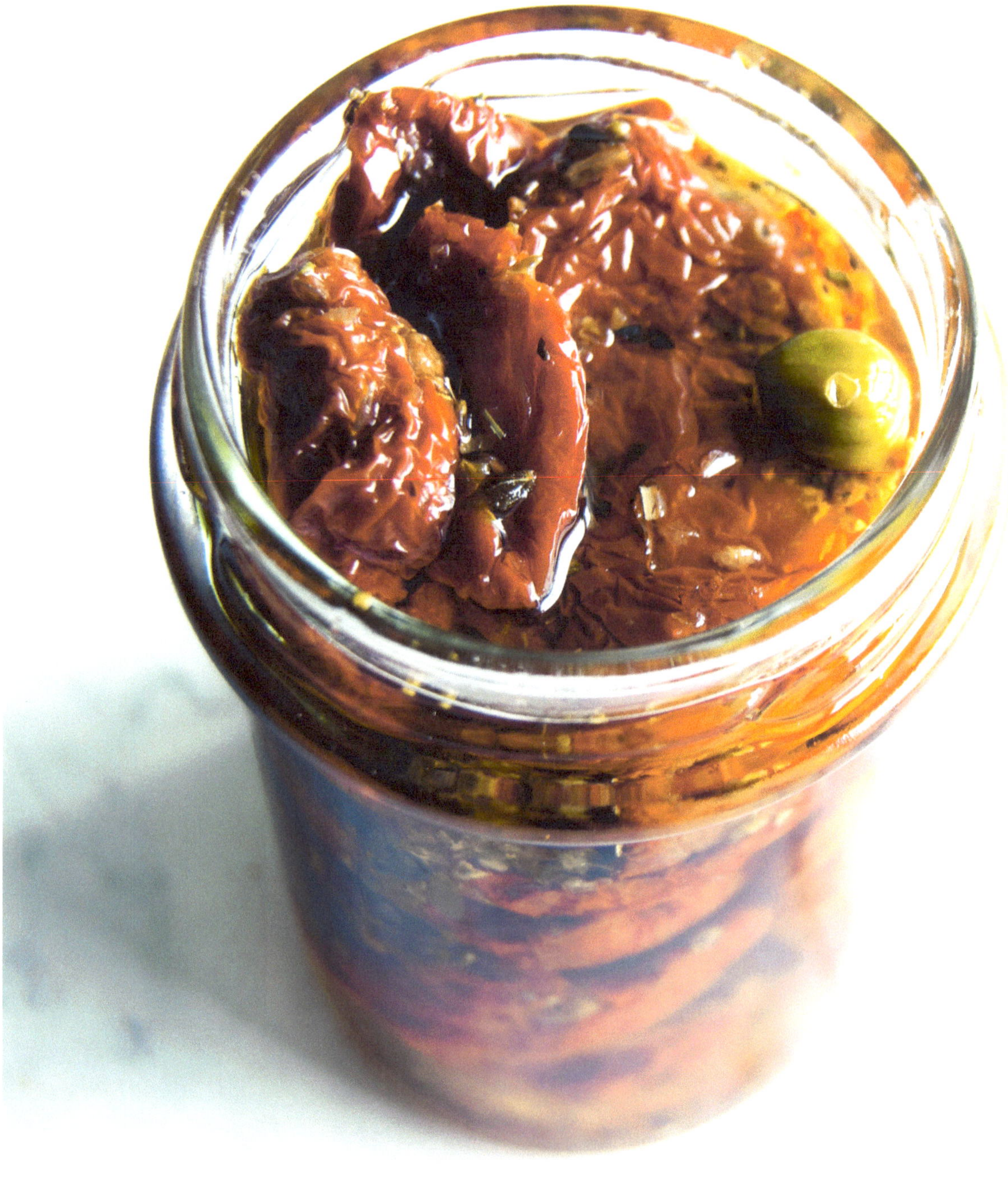

HOME STYLE SUNDRIED TOMATOES

Yield: 4

Ingredients

6 large tomatoes
1/2 tsp sea salt
2 tbsp olive oil
1/2 tsp thyme
1/8 tsp chili
1/2 tsp garlic
1 tbsp pickled capers

Line a dehydrator sheet with parchment paper. Set aside. Cut the tomatoes into quarters, remove the core and discard. Scoop out the seeds and as much tomato pulp as possible.

Transfer the tomato quarters to a large mixing bowl. Sprinkle with the salt, mix and let it sit 5-10 minutes. Tomatoes will release some of their juice, drain them. Add the oil, oregano, capers and thyme and stir to coat.

Place the tomato quarters cut-side up on the prepared baking sheet, making sure the tomatoes don't touch each other.

Dehydrate for about 12 hours, or until the tomatoes have reduced in size. Let cool completely. Place the dried tomatoes in a glass container and cover with olive oil. Dried tomatoes stored in oil will keep for up to 6 weeks in the refrigerator.

CAULIFLOWER PECAN CURRY PATE

Ingredients

2 cups raw pecans
1 cup cauliflower florets
1 tbsp curry powder
1 tbsp fresh dill chopped
1-2 tbsp lemon juice
1 tsp pink himalayan salt

Instructions

Place pecans and cauliflower into the food processor, mix on high speed until puree.
Place all remaining ingredients and combine together. Give it a good toss and transfer in a glass jar. Serve with raw crackers.

ITALIAN PATE

Ingredients

1 cup cashews or almonds soaked
1/2 cup home style sundried tomatoes
1 large red bell pepper
2 tbsp olive oil
2 tbsp lemon juice
1/2 cup kalamata olives
15 g fresh basil
1/2 tsp pink himalayan salt

Instructions

Place the sundried tomatoes into the food processor mix until you get smooth texture, add little water if you need.
Add all the remaining ingredients and mix until smooth.
Transfer in a bowl, serve with raw crackers.

CAULIFLOWER OLIVE TAPENADE

Ingredients

4 cups califlower florets
1 cup pitted kalamata olives
2 tbsp capers
3 tbsp olive oil
2 garlic cloves
2 tbsp fresh lemon juice
1 tbsp fresh thyme chopped
1 tbsp fresh parsley chopped
Salt and pepper to taste

Instructions

Place the cauliflower florets in a food processor , pulse until finer texture. Transfer to a bowl. Add olives, capers, garlic, olive oil, lemon juice, thyme, parsley, salt and black pepper. Pulse until combined and chopped small pieces. Pulse a few more times if you'd like to make olives into a paste. Add olive mixture to the cauliflower. Stir to combine, add more salt and olive oil of needed.

SPINACH SPIRULINA PATE

Ingredients

1/2 cup raw cashews or almonds
3 cups spinach
2-3 tbsp water
1 tbsp olive oil
1 tsp salt
1 tsp spirulina
1/4 tsp cayenne

Instructions

Place all the ingredients in a food processor.
Blend until everything combined well.
Transfer mixture in a bowl. Serve with the raw bread, crackers or enjoy on the top of your salad.

AVOCADO RANCH DRESSING

Ingredients

2 ripe avocados (200 g)peeled and core removed
100 g cashew yogurt
3 tbsp lemon juice
2 tbsp olive oil
3 tbsp fresh dill chopped
1 tbsp green olive chopped
3-4 tbsp water to thin as needed
2 garlic cloves minced
Salt and pepper to taste

Instructions

Place all ingredients in a blender and blend until smooth.
If you like it thicker, add less water. If you like it thinner, add more water.

This Avocado Ranch Dressing is a healthier take on the classic salad dressing. Avocado is a fantastic base for dressing and dips. It creates a silky, creamy consistency and the addition of fresh dill and chives add so much flavor! Perfect as a dip, a top salads, and more!

JACK SPINACH DIP

Ingredients

250 g baby spinach leaves
1/2 cup young jack fruit meat
100 g red onion thinly diced
70 ml filtered water
1 tbsp lemon juice
130 g raw almonds soaked
2 tbsp nutritional yeast
2 small garlic cloves minced
3 tbsp olive oil
1 tsp pink himalayan salt

Instructions

Chop your spinach and red onion, place in a large bowl. Set aside.
Add all the remaining ingredients to your blender expect olive oil , mix on high speed until smooth.
Transfer mixture into the large bowl with spinach and onion.
Toss together. Drizzle with olive oil.
Chill for 2 hours to increase the dips thickness. Garnish with chopped spring onions and red bell pepper if desired.
Consume within 2 days.

ARTICHOKE PATE

Ingredients

1 cup artichoke hearts
1 cup spinach leaves
1 cup nuts of your choice
1 cup water
2 garlic cloves minced
2 tbsp olive oil
3 tbsp lemon juice
A pinch cayenne
Salt to taste

Instructions

Place the artichoke hearts in a food processor, mix until chunky. Depending on preference, this may be more or less – I like an almost smooth texture. Add all remaining ingredients. Stir everything together. Let marinate in the fridge for at least an hour, and serve with raw crackers.

LEMON GARLIC AIOLI

Ingredients

1 cup young coconut meat or cashews
1/2 cup filtered water
2 tbsp olive oil
2 tbsp lemon juice
2 garlic cloves minced
1 tsp salt
1/2 tsp onion powder
1/2 tsp coconut vinegar

Instructions

Throw all of the ingredients into your blender, and blast on high for 30 to 60 seconds until smooth and creamy.

GREEN OLIVE SALSA

Ingredients

1 cup green olives

1 cup tomatoes

1/2 cup fresh fennel chopped

10 g fresh thyme

1 tbsp lemon juice

1 tbsp olive oil

1/2 tsp pink himalayan salt

1 medium cucumber

Instructions

Chop ingredients into small chunks, stir together in a bowl. Chill and serve with raw breads.

ZERO WASTE ALMOND CHUTNEY

Ingredients

1/2 cup almond pulp (from the almond milk pulps)

1 medium apple

1 orange peeled

2 tbsp dried raisins

2 tbsp lemon juice

1 tbsp fresh basil

A pinch cinnamon

Salt to taste

Instructions

Blend all ingredients until slightly chunky. This recipe is wonderful to use pulps when you make homemade almond milk. Keep the pulps in the freezer and use when needed.

TAMARIND GINGER DRESSING

Ingredients

4 fresh tamarind peeled seeds removed
3 fresh sukkari dates seeds removed
1 tbsp balsamic without sugar
2 tbsp fresh chopped parsley
1 tsp red chili flakes
4 g grated ginger
Juice of 1 lemon
Salt and pepper to taste

Instructions

Place the tamarind, dates, balsamic, ginger, chili, salt, pepper and lemon in your blender. Blend until you get a smooth paste. If you need add 1 tbsp water to thin. Pour mixture in a bowl, add the chopped parsley. Stir well. Serve with shredded carrots, salads, buddha bowls or whatever you like. This sauce tastes heavenly and goes well especially with the raw root vegetables. Make sure you slice the root veggies very thinly with the mandolin slicer to get the best taste.

CARROT RED PEPPER DRESSING

Ingredients

1 medium carrot shredded
1 large red bell pepper or capsicum
1 large tomato chopped
2 garlic cloves minced
2 g ginger finely grated
1 tsp red pepper flakes
1/2 tsp salt
1/4 tsp ground bay leaf

Instructions

Throw all of the ingredients into your blender, and blast on high for 30 to 60 seconds until smooth and creamy. Serve with your salads, sprouted quinoa or other grains of your choice.

COCONUT YOGURT

Ingredients

1 can full fat coconut milk

2 capsules of probiotic

Instructions

Open your coconut milk can and scoop out the solid cream. Depending how thick you like your yogurt, add more or none of the coconut water.

Place coconut milk in a clean jar or glass container. Stir the milk to combine, then take your probiotic capsules, open them up and add the contents to the milk.

Stir in the probiotics using a wooden spoon. Cover the jar with a clean cheese cloth or thin dishtowel, tighten with an elastic band and leave to sit on the counter for 24-48 hours (depending how warm your house is). Keep away from direct sunlight. It usually takes about 24 hours. You can give it a taste during the process, to make sure when your yogurt is done - look for the distinctive tangy yogurt taste.

Once done, place a lid on your container and place the yogurt in fridge for a couple of hours to thicken and firm. Keep refrigerated and consume in a couple of days.

APPLE CARAMEL DIP

Ingredients

4 large medjool dates
1 tsp apple cider vinegar
A pinch licorice salt
1 tbsp coconut oil melted
1 tbsp maple syrup
110 ml fresh apple juice
Thinly sliced apples to serve

Instructions

Place dates, coconut oil in the food processor. Mix on high speed until you get puree.

Place the remaining caramel ingredients in a blender jar and pour apple cider over the top. Blend on high until silky and smooth.

Transfer to serving dish, let cool to room temperature and serve with sliced apples.

APPLE MUSTARD DRESSING

Ingredients

1 cup red apples chopped
1 tbsp dijon mustard
2 garlic cloves minced
2 tbsp coconut vinegar or apple cider
1/2 cup water
4 fresh black mission figs

Instructions

Place all the ingredients in the Blendtec twister jar, blend until you achieve a smooth and creamy consistency. Transfer dressing in a weck jar. Use with your salads or as dip sauce with fruits.

Storage: This dressing can be kept in the refrigerator for 3-4 days.

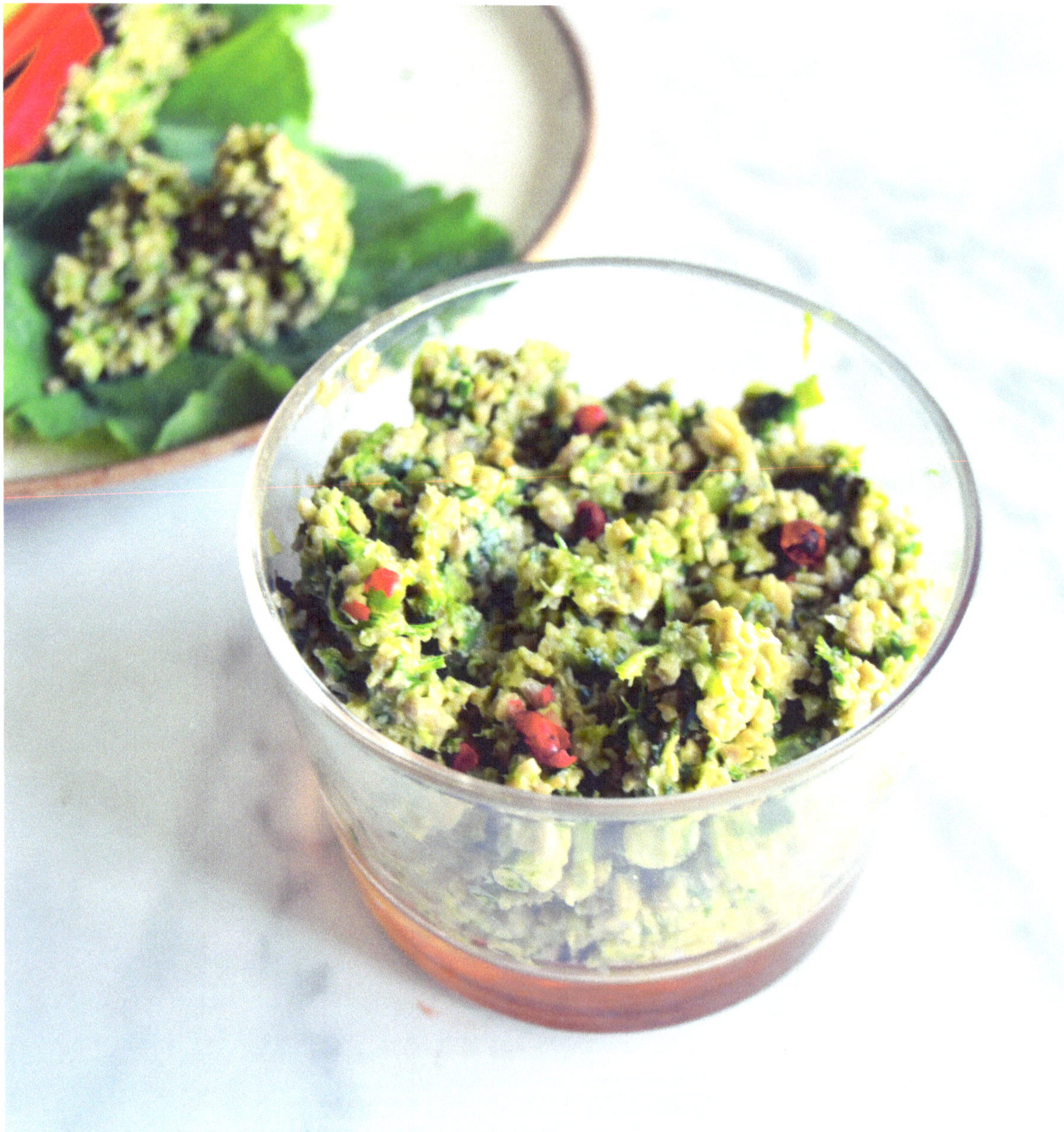

SUNFLOWER SEED PATE

Yield: 2 person

Ingredients

115 g raw sunflower seeds
A handful of fresh dill
2 medium celery stalks chopped
3-4 springs of green onions
1/2 tsp dulse flakes
1/2 tsp wakame flakes
1/2 tsp garlic powder
4-5 tbsp lemon juice
1 tbsp coconut nectar
2 tbsp fresh parsley chopped
1/4 tsp chili powder
1/4 tsp pink himalayan salt

Place all ingredients except green onion and parsley into a food processor and process until combined and texture is like a pate. You don't want to leave the mixture too chunky if you are going to spread it onto raw wraps. But if you like silky smooth, process again.

Place pate into a bowl, add green onion and parsley and stir carefully until combined.

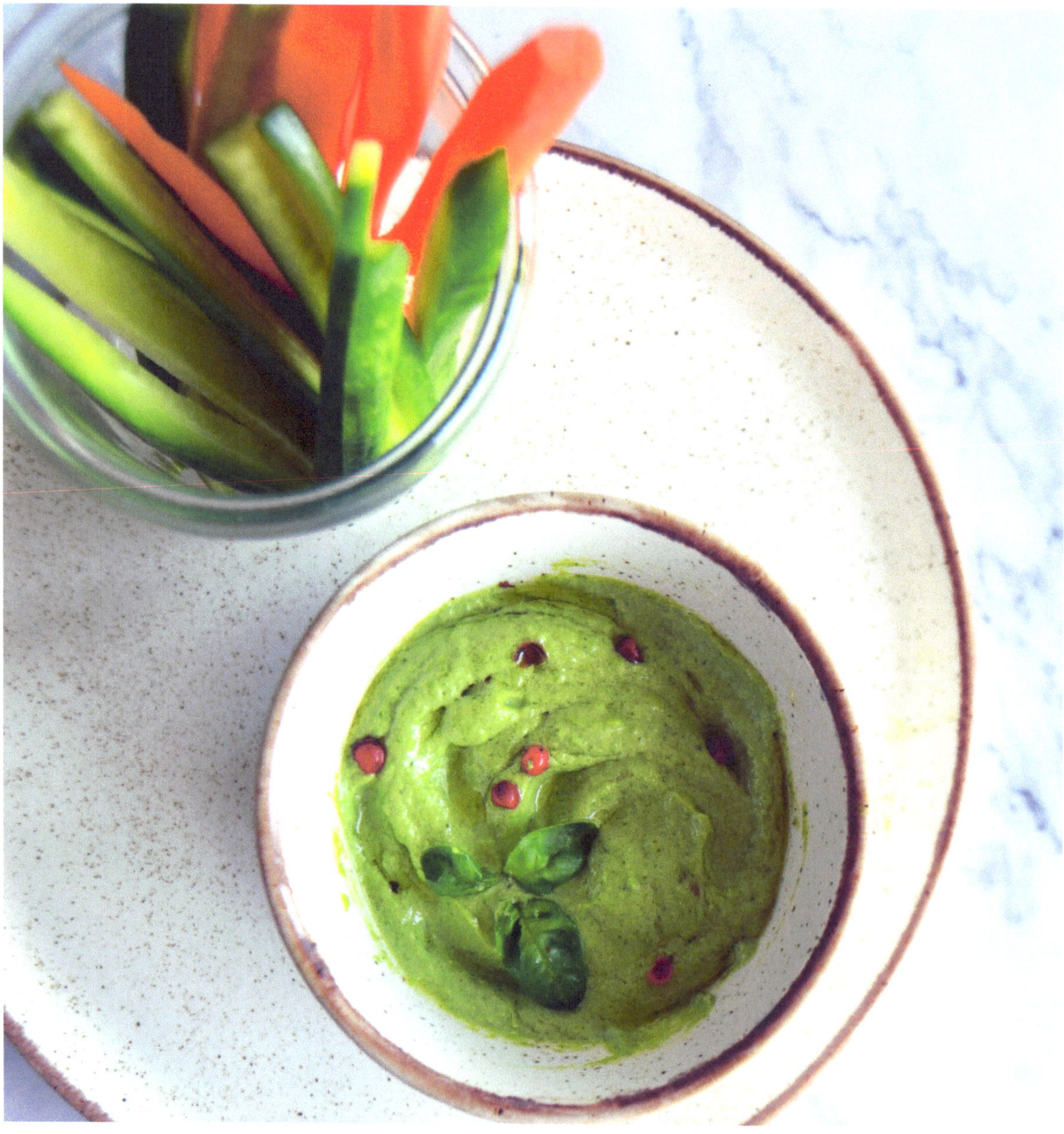

CREAMY BASIL DIP

Yield: 2 person

Ingredients

110 g raw cashews soaked
1/2 tsp garlic powder
45 g fresh basil
2 tbsp olive oil
3 tbsp lemon juice
1 tsp pink himalayan salt
50 ml filtered water
Cucumber, carrot to serve

Place all ingredients except cucumber and carrot in a high speed blender. Process until light and fluffy, scraping down the sides as necessary and adding an extra tablespoon of water if needed to thin the mixture.

Serve drizzled with extra olive oil and basil leaves alongside fresh cut vegetables.

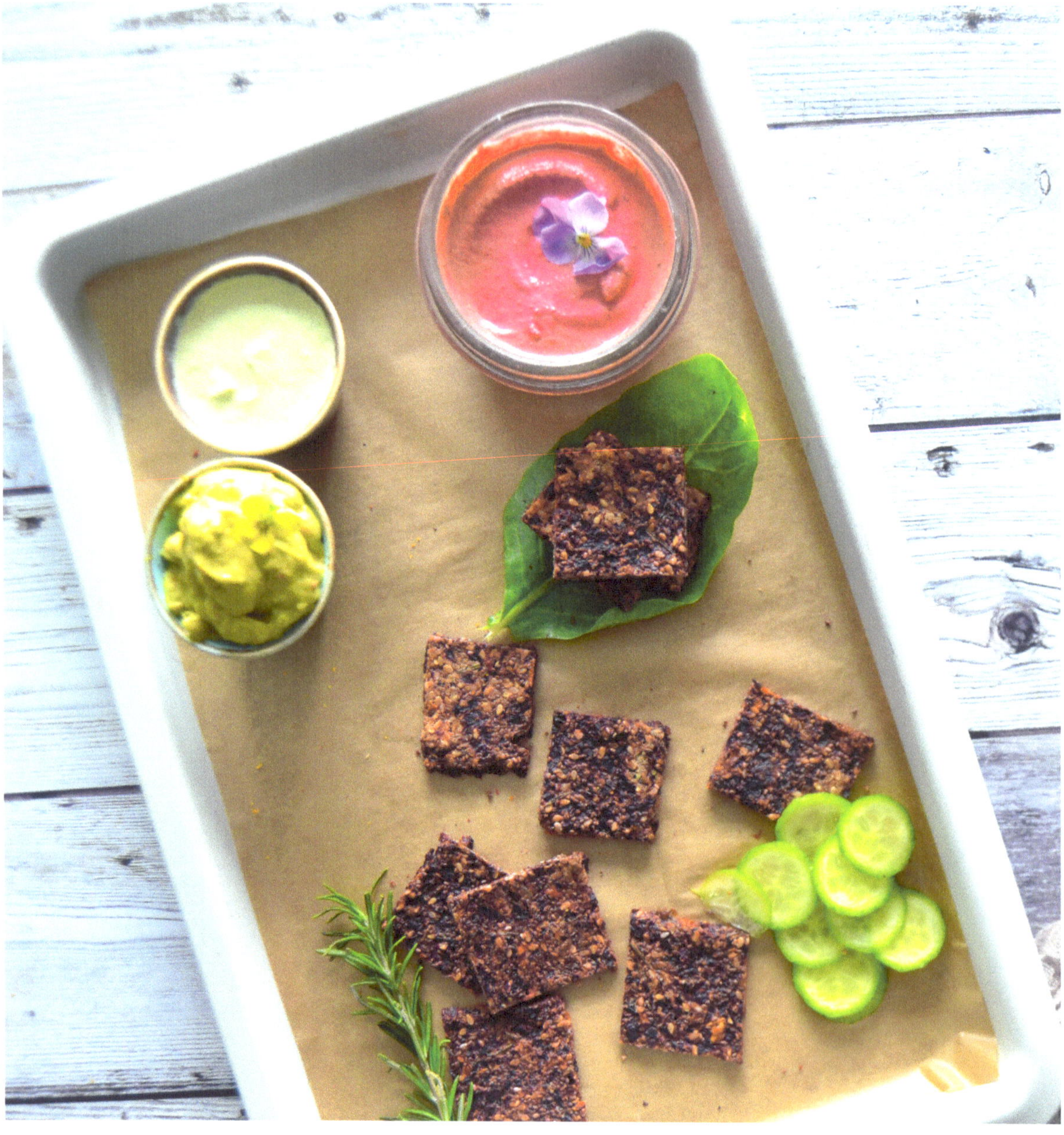

TZATZIKI SAUCE

Yield: 2 person

Ingrdients

150 g raw cashews
200 ml water
1 tsp garlic powder or 2 garlic cloves minced
3 tbsp lemon juice
1/2 tsp salt
1/2 tsp onion powder
1/8 tsp black pepper
60 g cucumber pulp removed water
3 tbsp fresh dill

Shred the cucumber and squeeze the excess water out through a fine mesh sieve and using your hands set aside.

Place cashews and water into the food processor, mix on high speed until smooth. Then add all remaining ingredients and mix again.

Transfer cashew cream mixture to a bowl and stir in the shredded cucumber and chopped dill. Refrigerate at least 1 hour before serving. To make pink , just add 1 tsp beet power and mix well. Serve with raw crackers or salad.

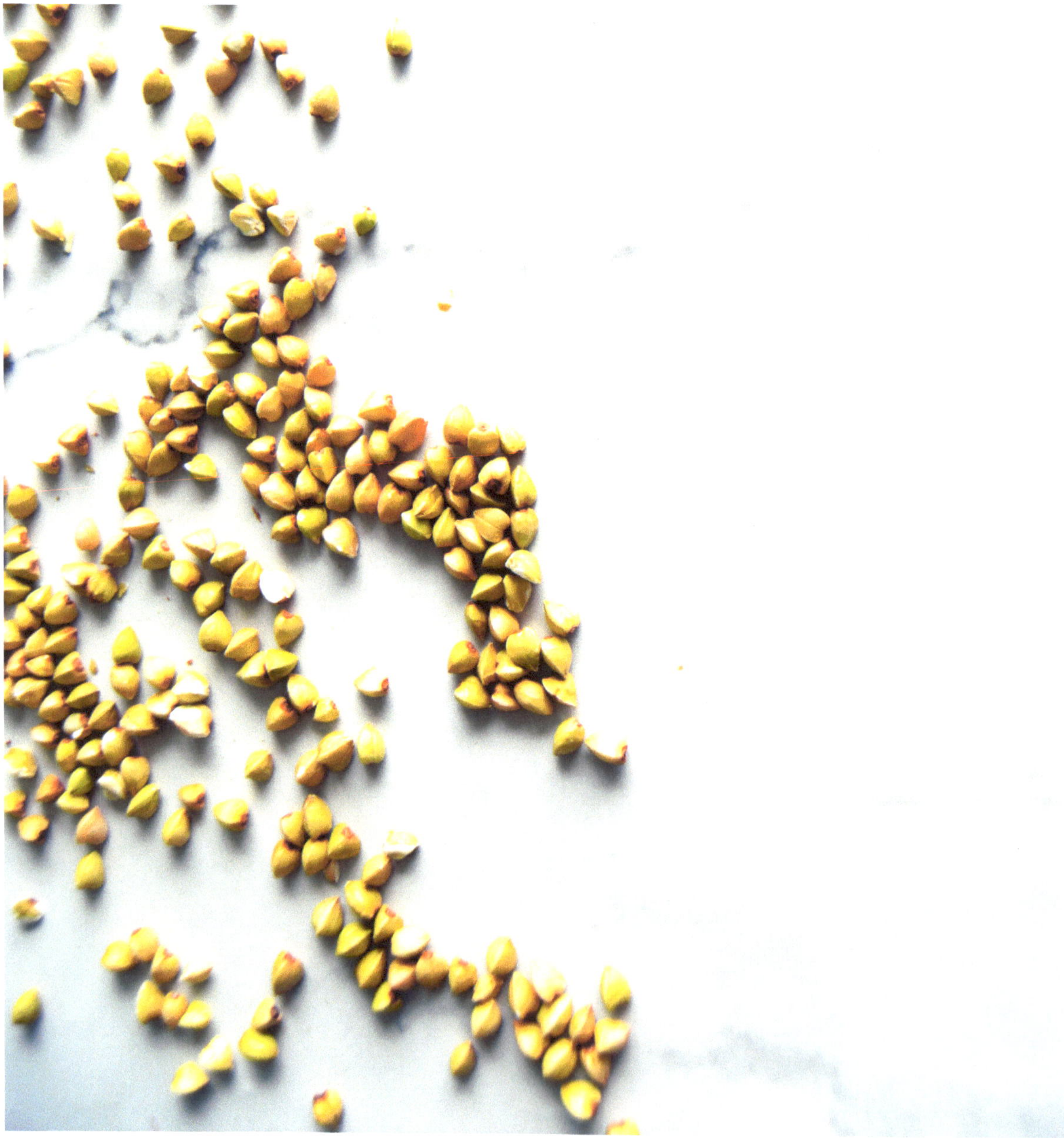

HOW TO MAKE BUCKINI

Buckinis are great addition to raw desserts, cereals , rawnolas, home-made muesli bars .
To consume raw, we need to activate them.

The reason you shouldn't be eating buckwheat groats raw without first activating them is due to the Phytic Acid in the grain. Phytic Acid binds to the nutrients within grains, legumes, nuts and seeds making them less available to us.

By soaking your grains and legumes you are significantly reducing the Phytic Acid content by activating the natural enzyme known as Phytase, which breaks down Phytic Acid and allows the nutrients contained in the food to become more bio-available, which basically means our bodies can absorb the nutrients and vitamins more readily.

To make:
Rinse your good quality, organic buckwheat groats under running water and pick out any bad bits. Put your washed buckwheat groats in a glass or ceramic bowl and cover with filtered, purified water to a good inch above the grain line. Add a tbsp of organic Apple Cider Vinegar – (this helps to further break down the Phytic Acid)

Soak for 6 hours minimum and 8 hours maximum. The water will become murky and slimy. Rinse well under running water. If you want to sprout them, repeat process 3 times a day.

Dehydrate them on a very low heat for 5-6 hours or until completely dry. Store in a glass jar.

"TAKE CARE OF YOUR BODY. IT'S THE ONLY PLACE YOU HAVE TO LIVE."

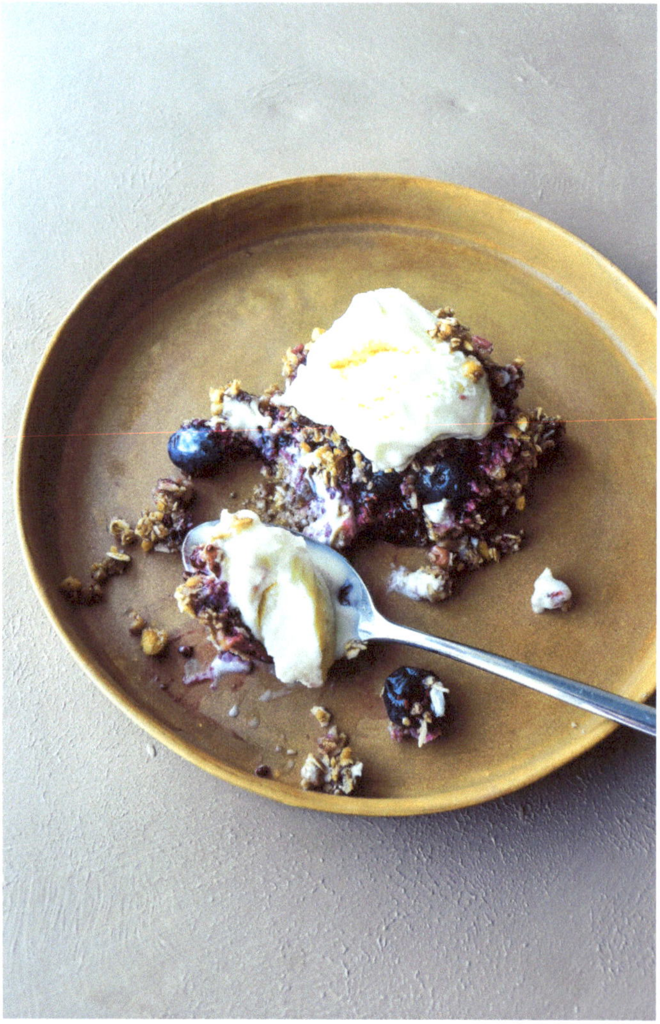

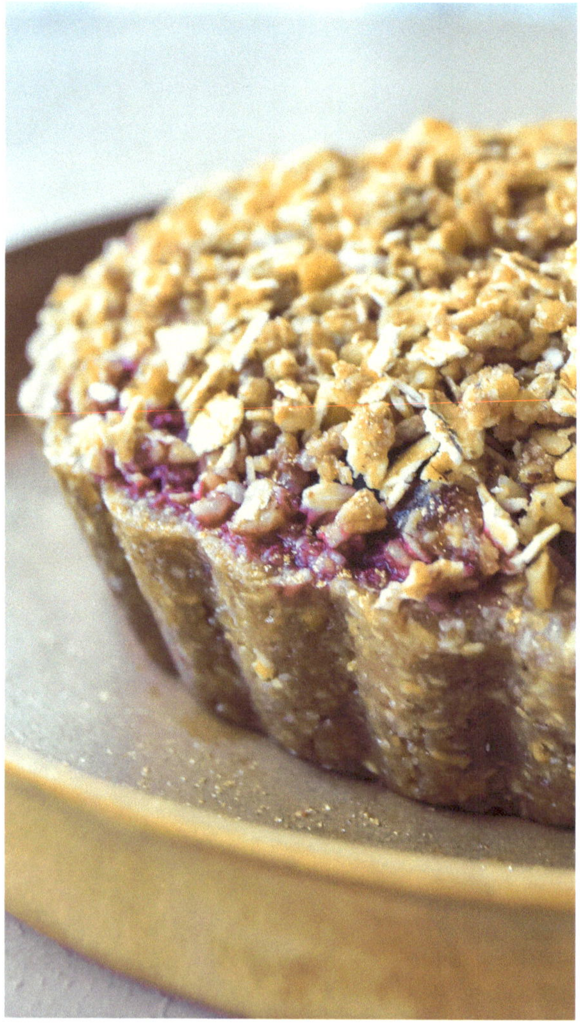

OAT WALNUT CRUMBLE

This raw crumble will please everyone, raw vegan, gluten free or otherwise. A rich, sticky crust is filled with a ginger bread spiced forest berries and a dollop of raw coconut ice cream for a balanced tangy finishing touch!

Yield: 15 round cake

Cake Ingredients

130 g sprouted rolled oats
65 g activated dehydrated walnut flour
65 g desiccated coconut
1 tbsp coconut flour
1 tbsp water
1 tbsp coconut butter
5 tbsp date paste
1/2 tsp vanilla bean powder
1 tsp cinnamon powder
1/2 tsp ginger powder
1/4 tsp cardamom
A pinch nutmeg
A pinch of licorice salt from Saltverk (or use pink himalayan salt)

Crumble

65 g sprouted rolled oats
65 g activated and dehydrated walnuts
1 tbsp coconut flour
2 tbsp date paste
2 medjool dates finely pitted
1 tbsp desiccated coconut
1 tbsp coconut butter
1/2 tsp cinnamon powder
1/4 tsp ginger powder
1/4 tsp cardamom
A pinch nutmeg
A pinch licorice salt (or pink himalayan)

oat walnut crumble continued

Filling Berry Jam

200 mixed forest berries of your choice (black-berry, blueberry, raspberry, lingonberry etc.)
65 g dried raisins soaked
2 tbsp chia seeds
1 tbsp maple syrup
1 tbsp psyllium husk powder
1 tsp orange zest
1 tbsp grated fresh ginger

Coconut Ice Cream

200g young coconut meat
130 ml oat milk
2 tbsp date paste
2 tbsp lemon juice
1 tbsp coconut butter

Place all the ingredients for the cake dough in a food processor and process until they combine into a dough. Once done, remove from the food processor and knead a little with your hands.

Place a parchment paper in a 15cm cake or pie tin and press the dough evenly into the tin. Make a nice about 1 – 1.5 cm edge along the shape. Set in the freezer for 10-15 minutes and make the jam.

Place berries and raisins in a bowl, add the rest of the ingredients for the filling berry jam. Mix well and let it sit while you are making the top crumble.

Roughly mix all ingredients except oats in the food processor. Add oatmeal and pulse shredded 1-2 times. Remove from the food processor.

Sprinkle the crumble on the berry jam layer. Let it sit for 1-2 hours in the fridge.

Place all the coconut ice cream ingredients into an ice cream maker, blend until you get silky smooth mixture. Then pour mixture in a rectangle mould. Freeze for 4-5 hours. Once done, using an ice cream scooper, scoop out and serve with your crumble cake.

ADVENT BREAKFAST BOWL

Yield: 2 person

Ingredients

110 g ripe avocados (1 ripe avocado, measured after deseeded)
160 g ripe bananas (1.5-2 small bananas measu-red after peeled)
1/4 cup unsweetened almond milk (2 pieces almond + 1/4 cup water blended together)
6 fresh dates pitted and chopped
2 tbsp raw almond butter
1 tsp orange or lemon zest plus more for garnish
1/2 cup pomegranate seeds to serve
1 tbsp pepitas to serve (raw pumpkin seeds)
A pinch of salt
1/4 tsp cinnamon powder
A pinch saffron

Crumb

1/4 cup raisins soaked and drained
1 cup almond butter
2 tbsp sprouted oat flour
1 tbsp sprouted buckwheat flour
1.5 tbsp maple syrup
1/4 tsp cinnamon
A pinch saffron
A pinch cardamom
A pinch salt

In a blender or food processor combine avocados, bananas and plant milk. Blend until smooth, adding more milk if needed to reach desired consistency.

Add the rest of the ingredients and blend until smooth.

Spoon into jars or serving dishes. Cover and chill at least 4 hours.

To serve, top with pomegranate seeds, pepitas, advent crumble. If desired, garnish with additional orange zest.

To make advent crumb, add the soaked and drained raisins in a food processor, add the almond butter and maple syrup. Blend together until smooth paste.

Then add the sprouted oat flour and buckwheat flour, a pinch of salt, cinnamon, saffron and cardamom. Process to combine together. We want them in crumble form, so do not mix so long otherwise may end with a sticky dough. If this happens, make crumble with your hands. Transfer mixture on a dehydrator sheet lined silicon paper. Dehydrate overnight or 8-10 hours until completely dried and crispy enough.
Serve on the top of your advent breakfast bowl or enjoy as a snack.

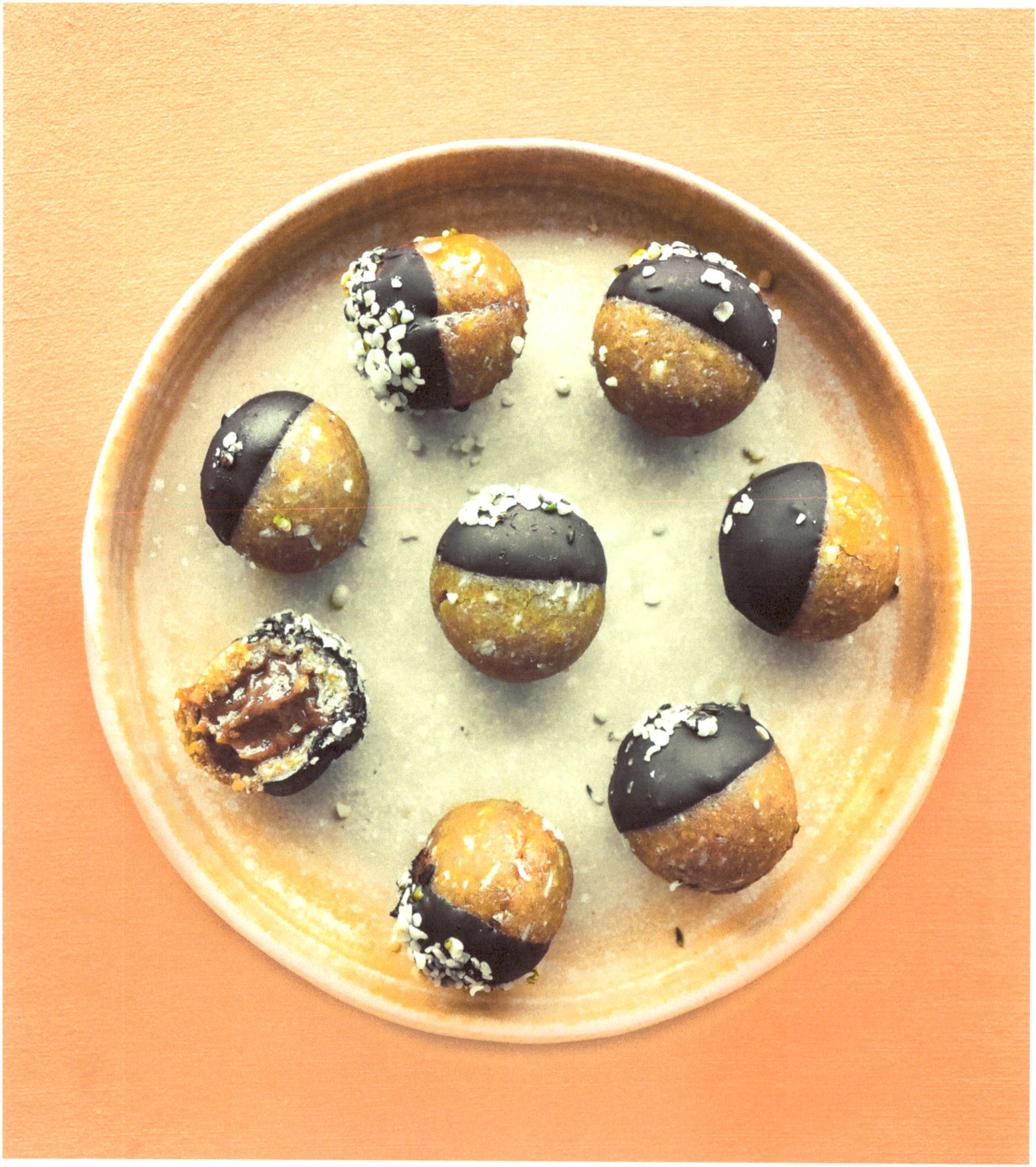

DATE CARAMEL FILLED BLISS BALLS

Yield: 3 cm 20 pieces (I used Pralinform hal-vklot mold from Pufz.se)

Crust

70 g sprouted rolled oats
50 g activated dehydrated almonds
15 g psyllium husk powder
15 g desiccated coconut
15 g almond butter
40 g maple syrup
60 ml plant milk or water
1/4 tsp pink himalayan salt

Caramel

85 g soft medjool dates (weight after seeds removed), soaked
30 g dried raisins, soaked
50 g almond butter
50 g maple
1 tsp cinnamon powder
1/4 tsp salt

Chocolate

60 g melted raw chocolate
Hemp hearts to decorate

Instructions

To make crust, place the oats, almonds in a high speed blender, process until you get powder. Then transfer mixture to a food processor, add the psyllium husk, desiccated coconut and salt, process until everything combined well. Add the almond butter, maple syrup and plant milk. Continue to mix until you get a dough-form. If it is too wet, add more desiccated coconut, if it is too dry, add extra plant milk, one tablespoon at a time.

Once done, take a teaspoon from the dough and fill the cavities of the mold. Use a teaspoon for each cavity. Press down with your hands and leave the middle of the cavities empty to fill with the caramel sauce.

Soak your raisins and dates in warm water for 20 minutes then strain and dry. Transfer to a high speed blender (I used Blendtec with twister jar.) Add the rest of the ingredients. Blend until everything combined well and you get a silky smooth caramel consistency.

Transfer mixture in a piping bag, alternatively you can use a teaspoon to fill the middle of the cavities.

Repeat the process for the rest. Put in the freezer for 30 minutes then, remove the cavities from the mold, combine each one with the other one to make a ball.

Using a bain marie method, melt the raw chocolate. Add 1/2 to 1 tsp chocolate (cover all or half of the top with chocolate). Sprinkle some hemp hearts over the chocolate. Freeze for 1 hour or keep in the refrigerator for 2-3 hours or until completely cooled. Then remove from the mold.

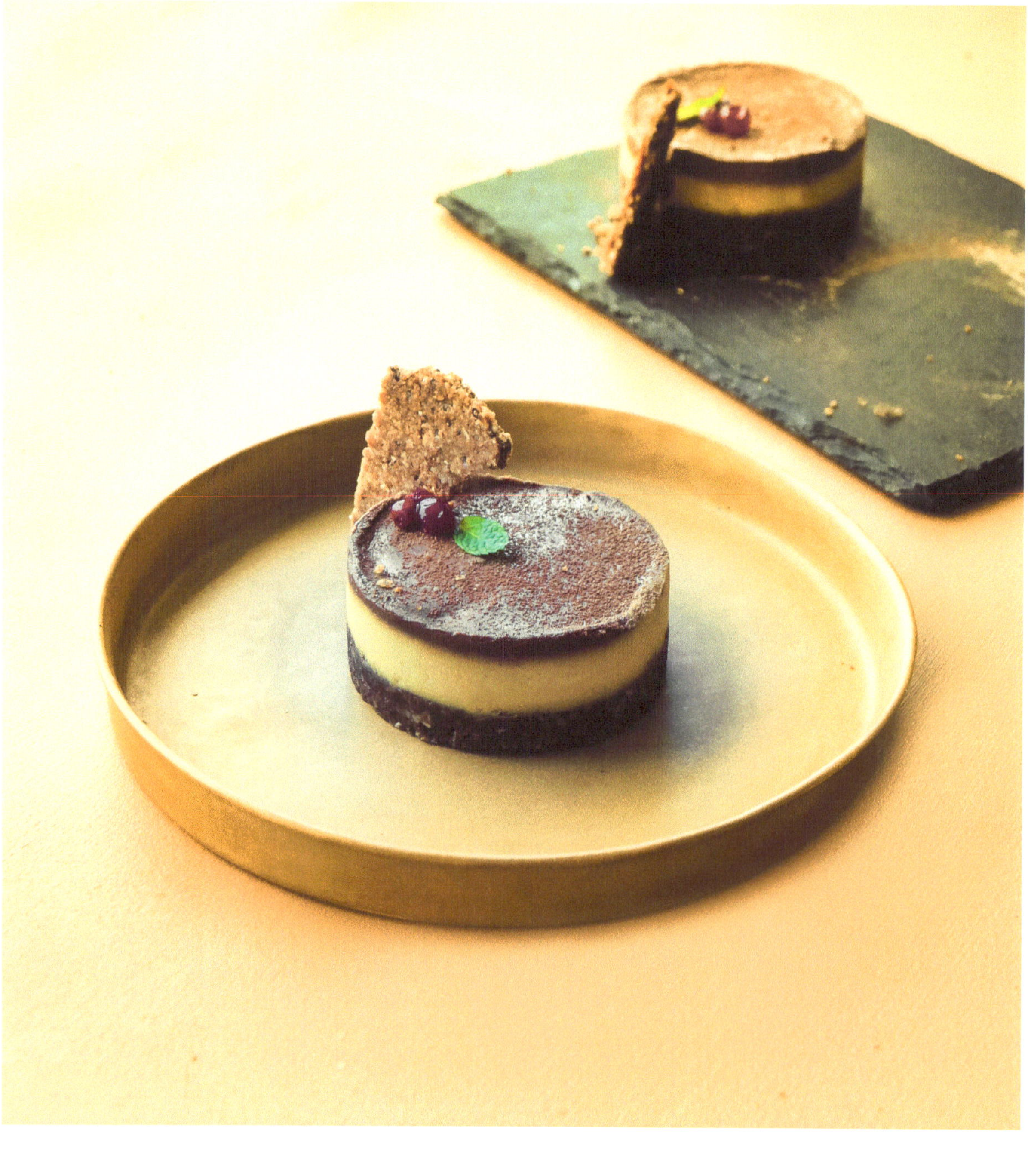

THREE LAYER RAW CHOCOLATE CAKE

Yield: 3 x 7 cm ring molds

Crust

20 g brazil nuts
20 g sprouted rolled oats
20 g hazelnuts
75 g medjool dates soaked strained
1 tbsp raw cacao
2 tbsp hazelnut butter
1/4 tsp pink himalayan salt

Cream

75 g young coconut meat or cashews, macadamias soaked
2 tbsp maple
2 tbsp lemon juice
1 tbsp cacao butter melted
1 tbsp coconut oil melted
2 tbsp coconut milk

Ganache

45 g raw cacao butter melted
3 tbsp maple syrup
3 tbsp almond milk
2 tbsp raw cacao powder

Place brazil nuts, rolled oats and hazelnuts into food processor. Process until you get fine powder.
Then add the raw cacao, soaked strained dates, hazelnut butter and salt. Mix until everyting combined well and you get a sticky dough.
Divide dough between 3 round moulds about 7 cm. Flatten out with the back of the spoon or handle of the mold if you have.
Place all the cream ingredients in a blender (with twister jar). Blend until smooth.
Pour the cream over the crusts. Freeze for 30 minutes.
Place all the ganache ingredients in your blender. Blend until everything combined well.
Pour the ganache over the cream. Dust some cacao. Freeze for 2 hours.
Once done, remove from the molds.
Serve with raw brittles, lingonberries or yoru favorite fruit.
To make brittle, roll out your favorite bliss ball recipe, dehydrate overnight until completely dried. Then break into shards. Enjoy alone or serve with the raw cakes.

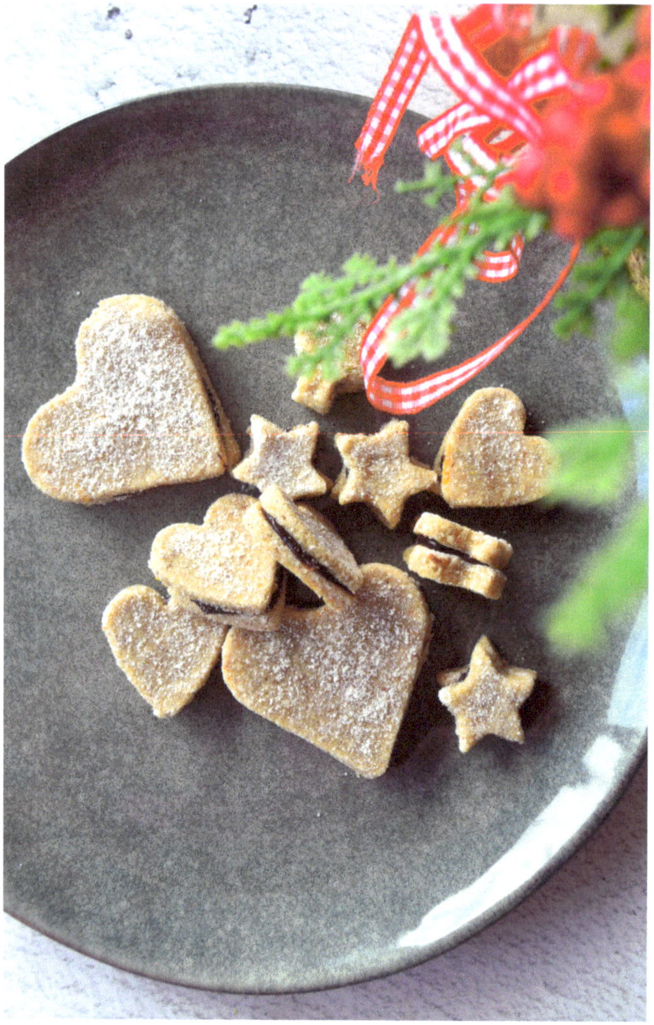

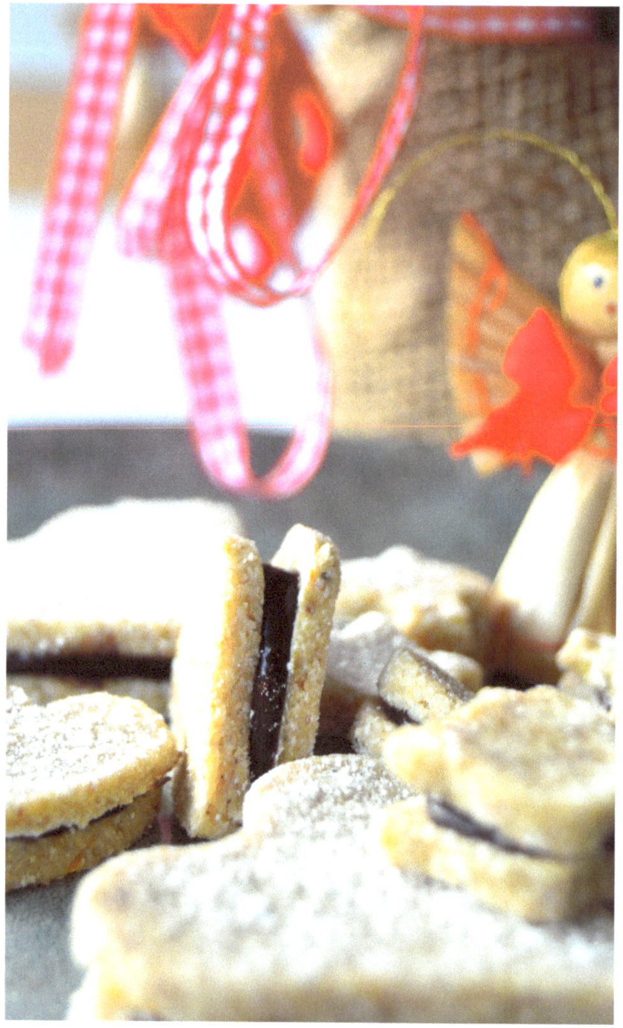

BUCKWHEAT COOKIES

Yield - 8-10 cookies

Ingredients
70g raw buckwheat
60g raw almond flour
2 tbsp coconut flour
60 g maple syrup
5g psyllium powder + 2 tbsp water
1 tbsp orange zest
1 tsp all spice, cinnamon, cardamom, ginger powder mixture
1 tsp vanilla powder
A pinch salt

Soak the raw buckwheats for 1 hour then rinse and allow to sprout for 10-12 hours or overnight.

Once they are sprouted, rinse well and transfer to your food processor, blend well for 2-3 minutes.

Then add the almond flour, coconut flour, salt, vanilla, spice mixture, blend again until well combined.
Add the maple syrup , psyllium powder and water. Blend on low speed until combined together.

Using your hands, mix it all up and form into a ball.
Roll it out between two pieces of parchment paper to about ¼ inch thickness.
Using your favorite cutter, cut them into hearts, Christmas tree, stars, Santa or whatever you want.
Repeat this process until all dough is used.

Place the cookies into the dehydrator lined dehydrator sheets to dry at around 42-46°C for 8 hours.

When done, let them cool and then dip the sides in raw jam, avocado frosting or just keep them as is.

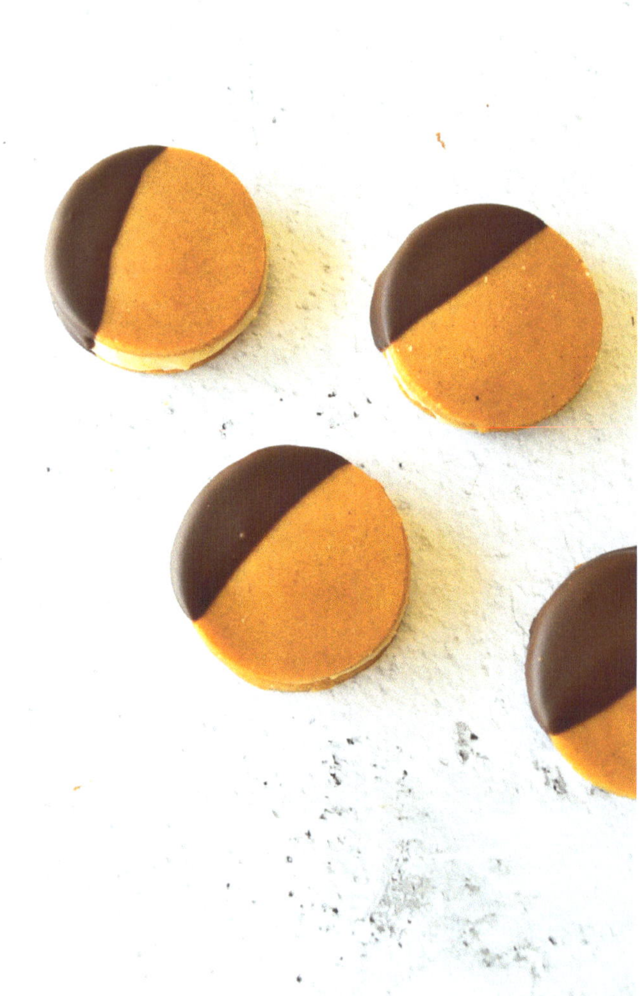

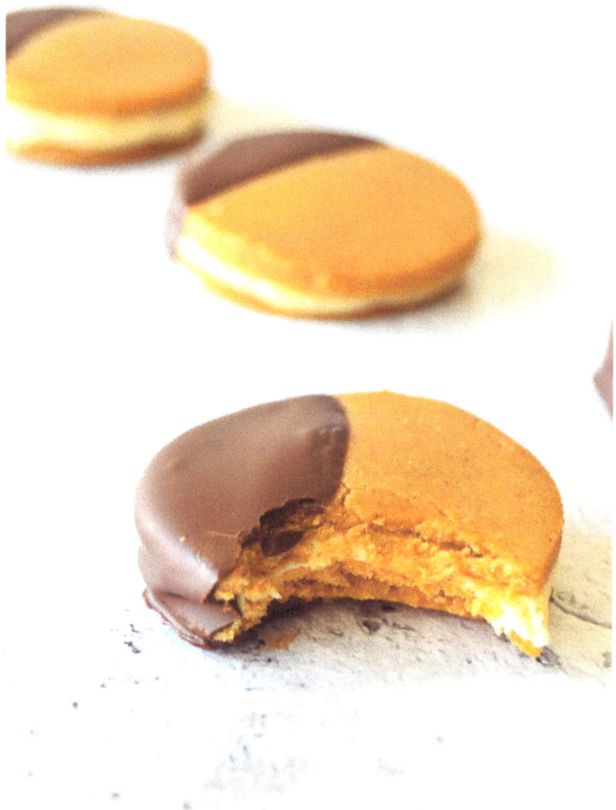

PEANUT BUTTER MACA COOKIES

Yield: 8-10 pieces

Ingredients
95 g gluten-free sprouted oat flour
25 g maca powder
90 g maple syrup
180 g raw peanut butter
1/2 tsp salt

Filling
70 g raw cashews or young coconut meat
1 tbsp lemon juice
4 soft dates pitted
2 tbsp coconut cream
1/2 tsp vanilla bean powder
1 tbsp + 1 tsp raw cacao butter melted

Topping
60 g raw chocolate melted

Place the sprouted oat flour, maca powder and salt in a high speed food processor, blend until combined well.
Add the peanut butter and maple, process to combine. You will get a nice smooth sticky dough. It can be easily shape.
If it is too wet, add a little bit more oat flour, one tablespoon at a time.
Transfer mixture between parchment papers. Using a rolling pin, roll out.
Using 5 cm round cookie cutter, cut the cookies.
Dehydrate the cookies for 12h at 46°C.
I love how they come out but if you don't have a dehydrator no worries, just re- frigerate them until set. They will still be delicious!
Meanwhile, transfer all the filling ingredients in a high speed blender (Blendtec with twister jar works great for small batches), blend until smooth cream.
Transfer mixture in the freezer for 15 minutes. Once chilled, it will be easier to work with.
Fill a pastry bag with the cream, pipe up your cookies. (Spread fillings if you don't have pastry bags.)
Using bain marie method, melt the chocolate. Dip your the half of your cookies in the chocolate. Transfer to a plate lined parchment paper. Let them cool at least two hours.
Keep them refrigerated in an airtight container up to 4 days.

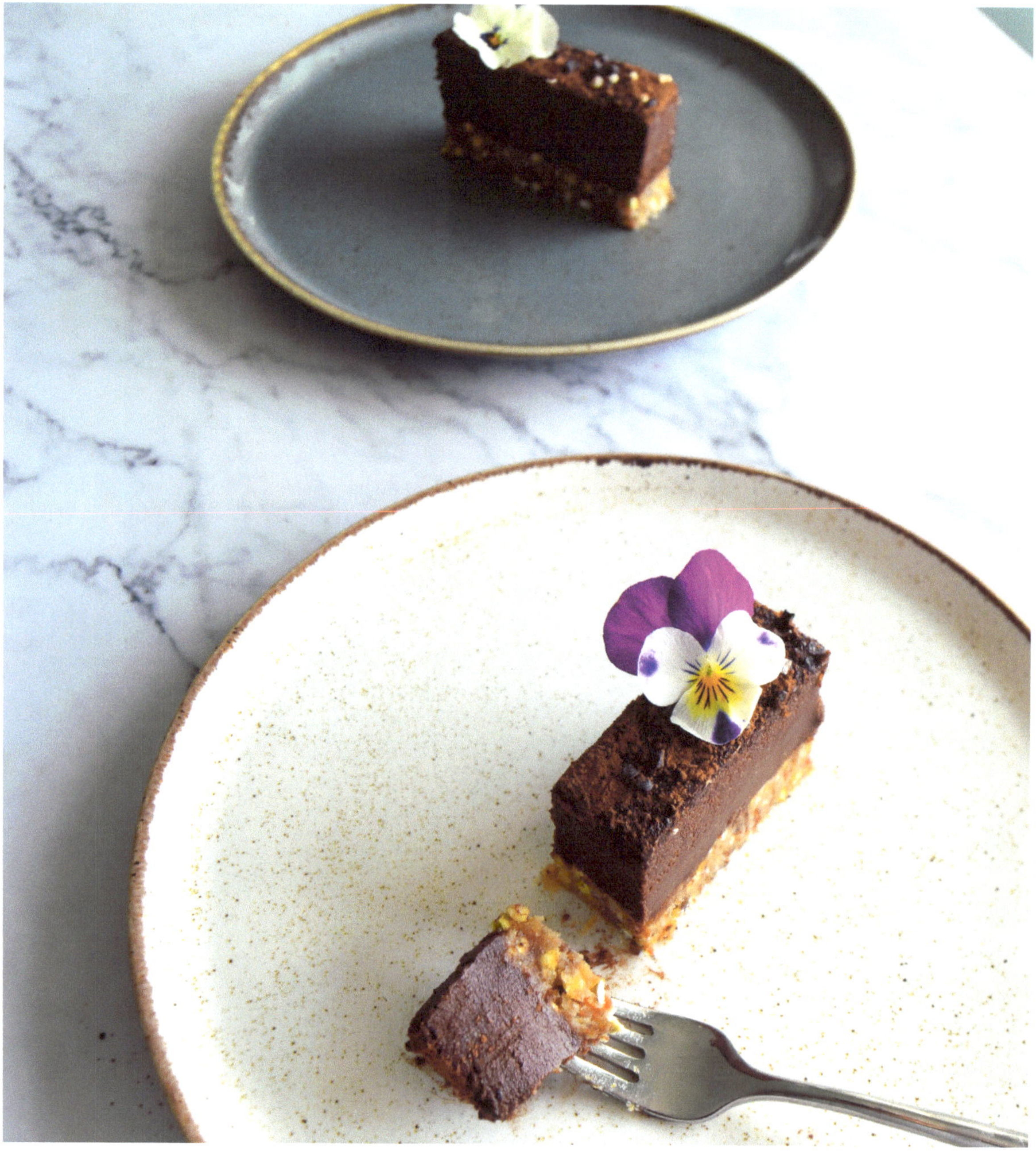

ORANGE FLAVOURED CHOCOLATE MOUSSE CAKE WITH CRUNCHY BUCKWHEAT CRUST

Yield: 6-7 slices

Crust

1/2 cup buckini (activated dehydrated buckwheat groats)
1/2 cup dates soaked and strained well
1/2 cup raw almonds
2 tbsp almond butter
1/4 tsp pink himalayan salt

Mousse

2 ripe avocados, skin and stone removed
1/2 cup (60 g) raw cacao
1/2 cup (125 ml) maple syrup
1/2 cup (125 ml) coconut cream
1/4 cup (60 ml) coconut oil
1 tsp vanilla bean extract
10 drops doTERRA wild orange essential oil
A pinch of salt

To make the crust, pulse almonds and buckinis in your food processor until they're in rough chunks.
Remove from the food processor. Set aside.

Process dates and almond butter in your food processor until fairly smooth and then add almonds back in along with salt. Pulse until combined.Press into a rectangle mold lined with parchment paper. Even out and pop in the freezer while you make the mousse.

To make the mousse, process avocado, coconut oil and coconut cream along with vanilla, wild orange essential oil.

Add raw cacao powder and salt and process until smooth.

Spread over the base and refrigerate until set for about 4 hours.

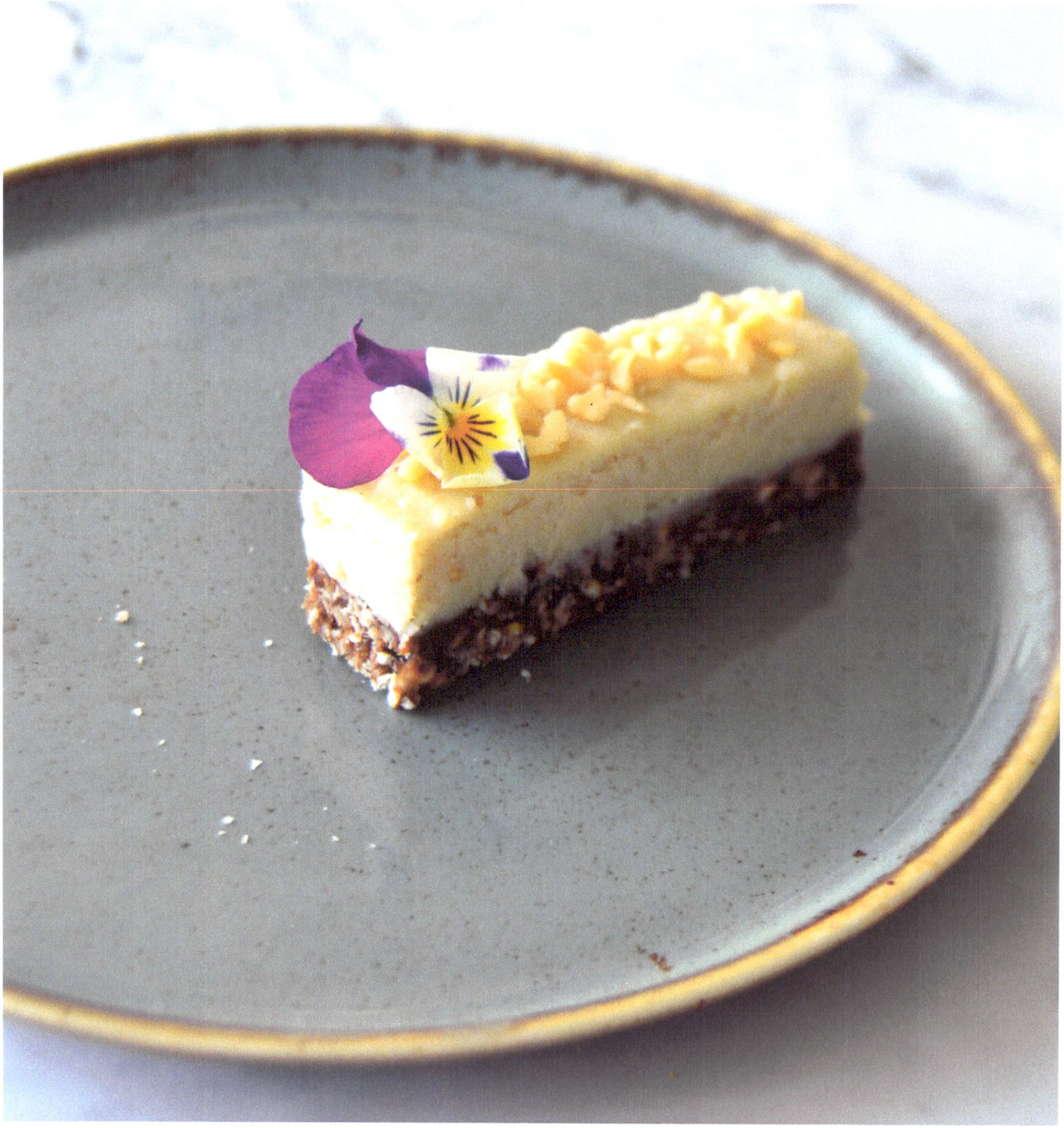

COCONUT LEMON CHEESECAKE

Yield: 6 slices

Crust

1/2 cup buckinis
1/2 cup raw almonds
1/2 cup dates soaked strained
2 tbsp coconut oil
2 tbsp raw cacao
1/4 tsp pink himalayan salt

Filling

1 cup raw cashews or macadamia
50 ml maple syrup
1/2 cup coconut cream
70 ml coconut oil
1 tsp vanilla bean cream
5 tbsp lemon juice

Pulse almonds and buckinis in your food processor until they're in rough chunks. Remove from the food processor. Process dates and melted coconut oil in your food processor until fairly smooth and then add almonds back in along with cacao powder and salt. Pulse until combined. Press into a pan with baking paper. Freeze while you make filling.

To make the smoothest cheesecake, you will need a high-speed blender. Process the soaked cashews, vanilla, coconut cream and melted coconut oil together with the lemon juice and maple syrup until completely smooth.

Remove crust pan from the freezer. Spread over the top of your base, add some crushed almonds on the top and leave to set in the freezer for 2 hours. Decorate with edible flowers and serve!

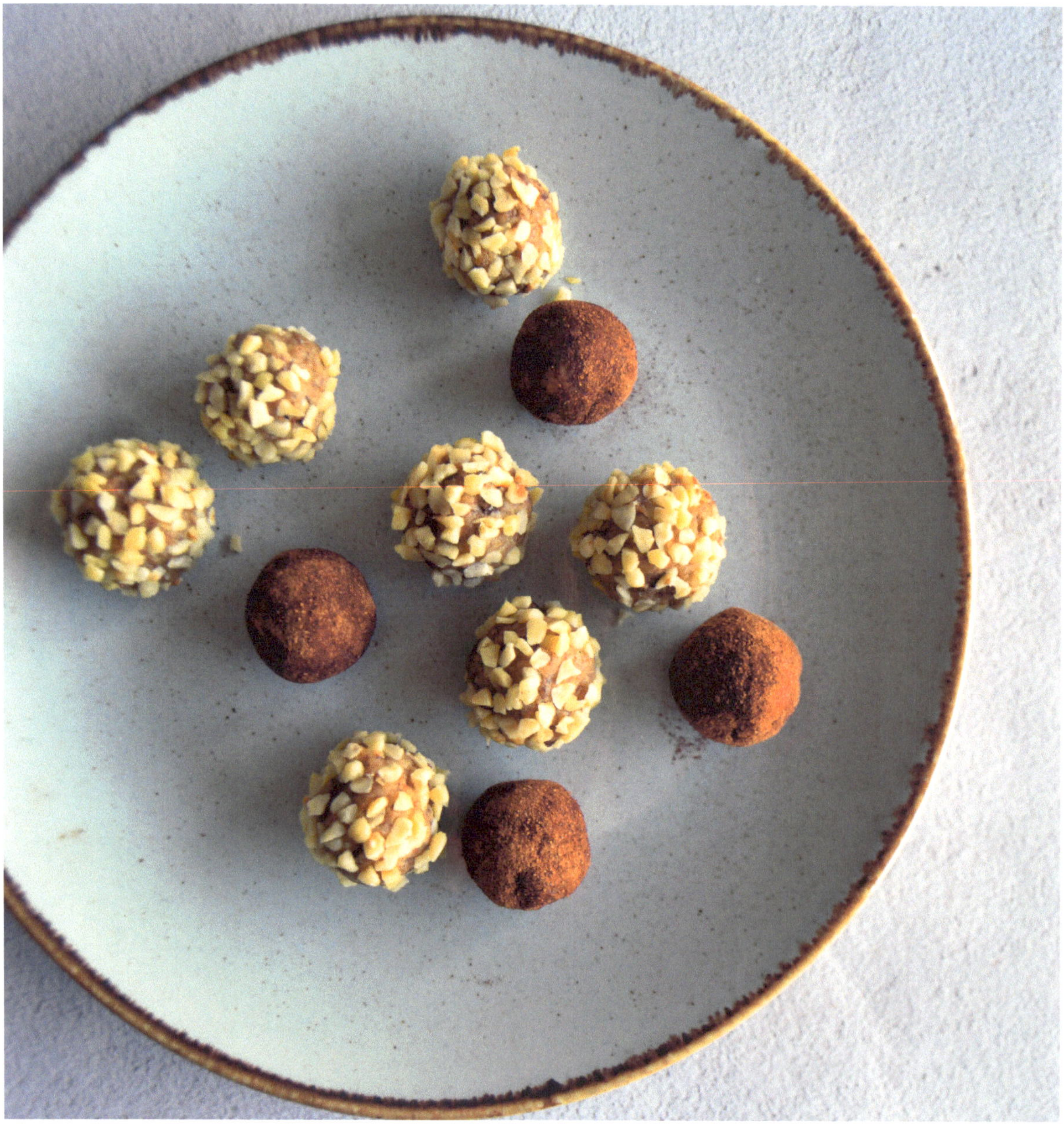

CINNAMON BALLS

Yield: 2 person

Ingredients

100 g sprouted rolled oats
125 g medjool dates soaked strained
1 tsp cinnamon
1/2 tsp cardamom
1/4 tsp clove powder
1/2 tsp ginger powder
2 tbsp raw cacao powder
2-3 tbsp plant milk
A pinch salt

Place the oats into the food processor mix on high until powdered. Then add dates and mix on high until sticky.

Add the rest of the ingredients, blend until everything combined well and you get a sticky dough.

Make small balls with your hands. Cover with raw cacao, cinnamon or crushed almonds of your choice.

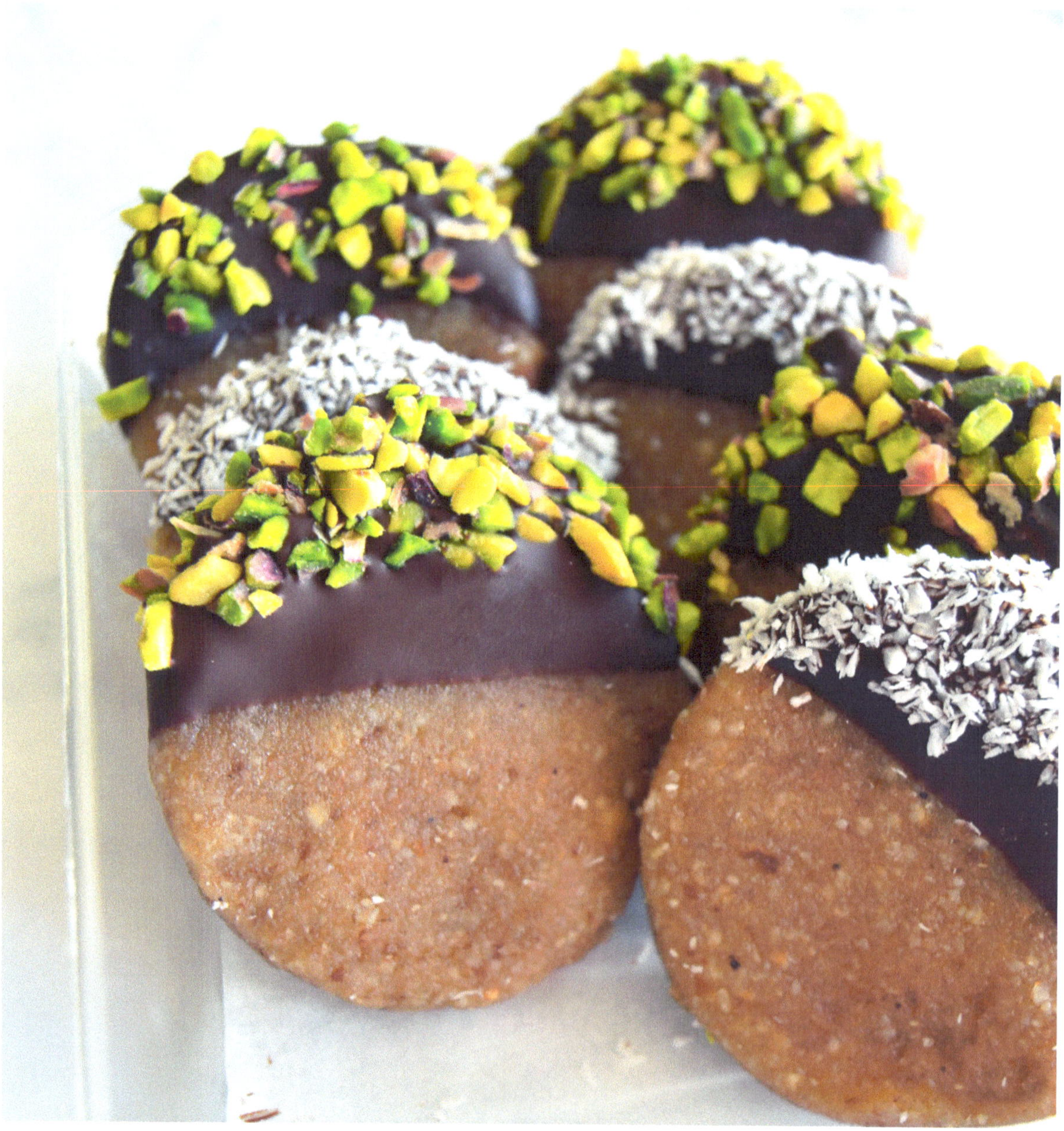

CHOCOLATE DIPPED RAW COOKIES

Yield: 2 person

Ingredients

120 g medjool dates
120 g activated raw cashews
100 g activated raw almonds
3 tbsp maple syrup
2 tbsp lemon juice
A pinch salt

140 g raw chocolate melted for dipping
10 drops wild orange essential oil
4-5 tbsp chopped pistachip for garnish
4-5 tbsp shredded coconut for garnish

Place the dates in your food processor, mix dates until they break into small pea-sized pieces. Add the almonds and cashews then process until well combined. Add the maple syrup. continue to process until dough comes together to form a ball. Continue processing until everything is well combined. Dough will be somewhat sticky but should still hold a shape. Scoop teaspoons of the 'dough' out and roll into balls. Place between baking paper and either using the palm of your hand or a rolling pin, roll flat. Place in the freezer for 30 minutes

Melt raw chocolate in a double boiler at 42°C, add the wild orange essential oil. Slowly mix until they are combined well. Transfer chocolate mix in a large bowl. It should be large enough to dip cookies easily.

Dip your cookies into the chocolate mix, allowing it to coat half of the cookie. Sprinkle chopped pistachios or shredded coconuts on the chocolate while it's still wet. Keep in refrigerator for several weeks.

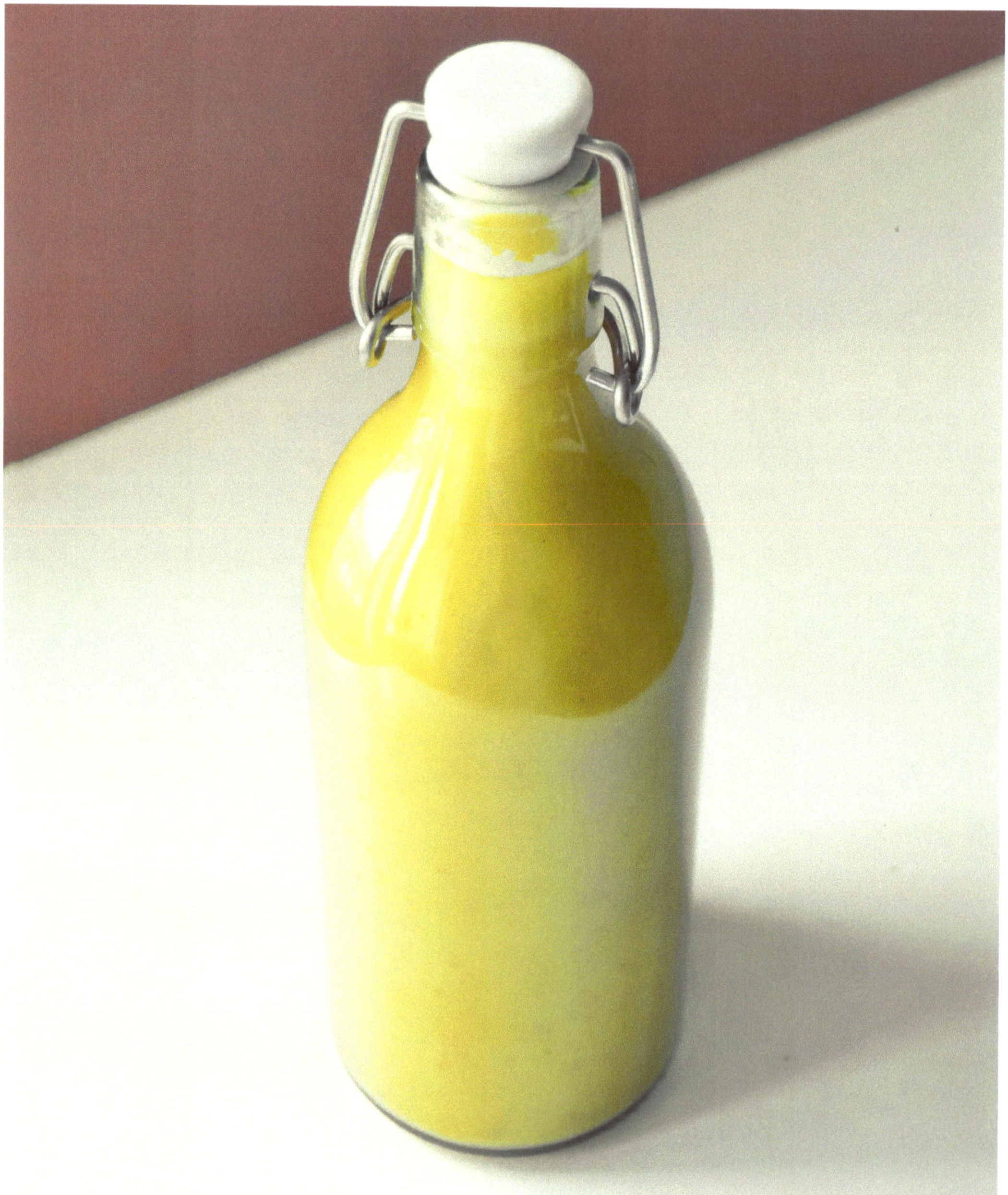

ST. LUCIA MILK

Yield: 2 person

Ingredients

2 cups filtered water
1/4 cup dried raisins
8 -10 raw almonds soaked
1/2 tsp cinnamon
A pinch dried saffron
A pinch cardamom powder
A pinch clove powder
A pinch salt

Soak almonds and dried raisins in warm water for 15 minutes, then strain and drain, transfer to a blender.
Add the filtered water, saffron, cinnamon, cardamom and salt.
Blend until you get smooth, yellow color milk.
Using a strainer, vegan milker or cheesecloth, strain the milk, remove the pulp.
Pour the milk in a 500 ml glass jar. Store in the refrigerator.
Enjoy!

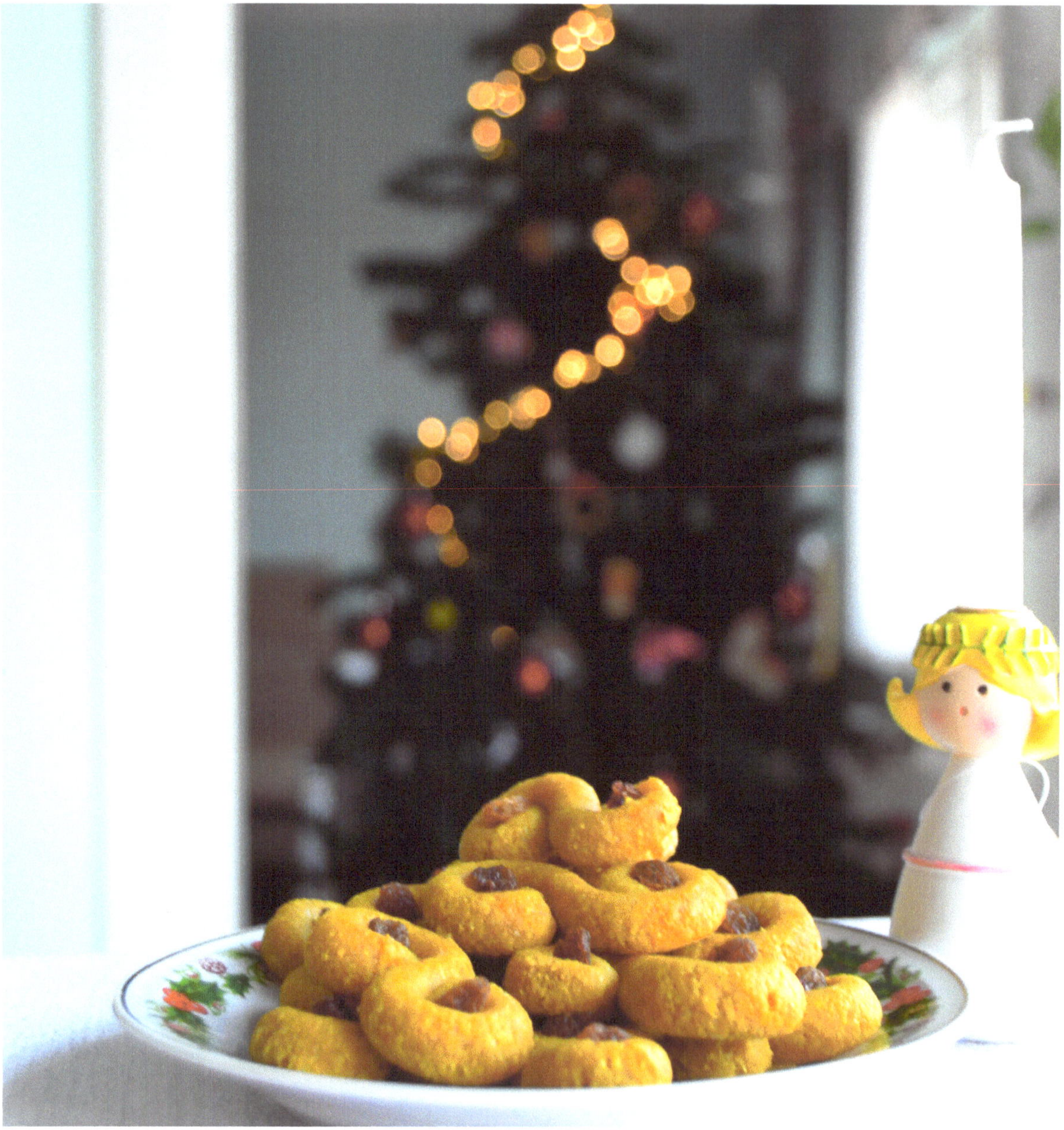

ST. LUCIA SAFFRON BUNS

Yield: 12-14 buns

Ingredients

90 g raw almonds
65 g sprouted raw sunflower seeds
65 g sprouted raw rolled oats
2-3 tablespoons maple syrup
2 tablespoons coconut sugar
1 tablespoon psyllium powder + 3 tablespoons water
0.2 g saffron + 1 teaspoon water + 1 teaspoon sesame oil
1/4 cup dried raisins for garnish

Stir the saffron in 1 teaspoon water and 1 teaspoon sesame oil in a small bowl. Set aside.

Mix water and psyllium.

Beat nuts and seeds into flour in a food processor or blendtec.

Pour in the rest of the ingredients and continue to run until the batter forms a ball.

Divide the dough into 12 pieces and roll out gently into saffron bun shape or balls.

Poke down raisins.

Dehydrate in the excalibur food dehydrator at 42 ° C for 12-14 hours until completely dried.

Tip: The aroma of saffron dissolves best in oil and its color best in water, so I used both to stir out the small straws.

Glad Lucia!

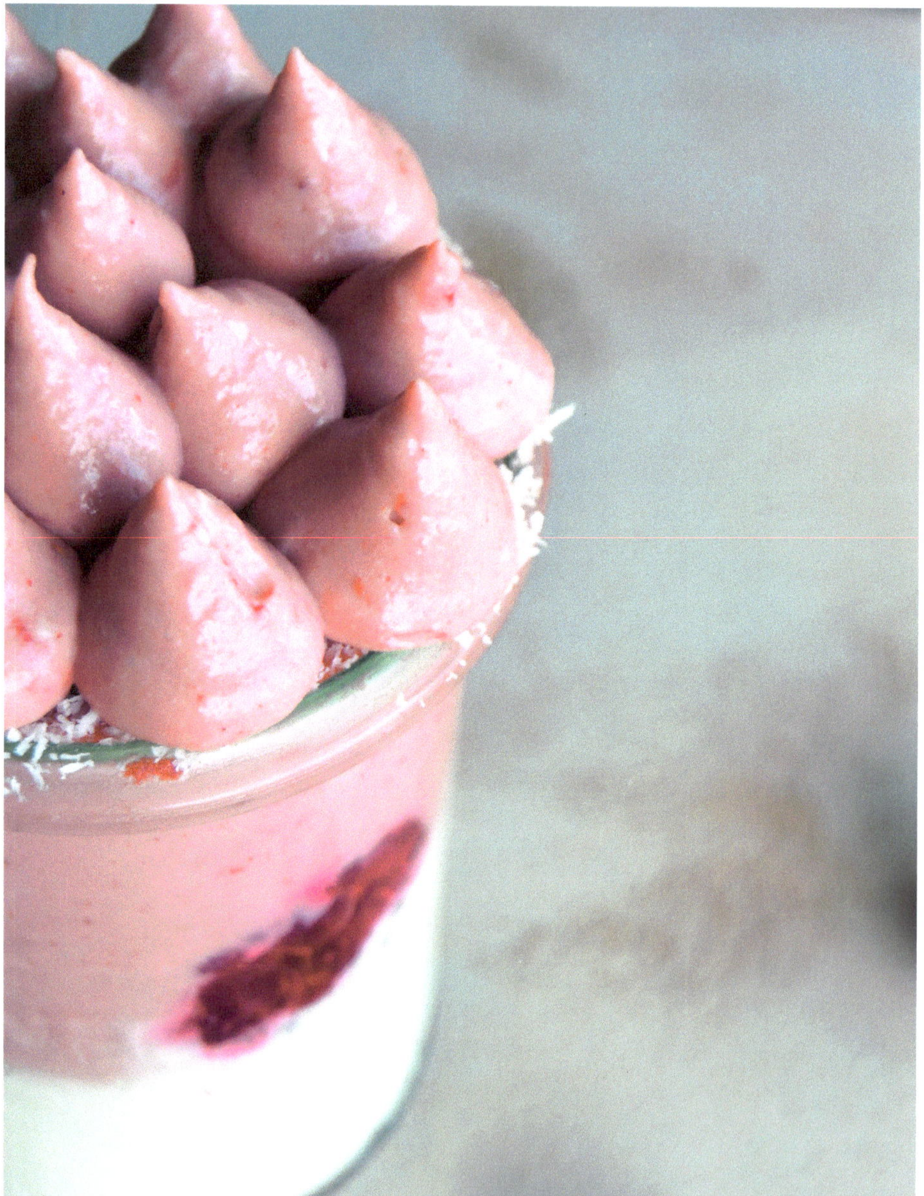

COCONUT STRAWBERRY PARFAIT

Yield: 2 jars of 160 ml each

Ingredients

2 cups young coconut meat
1 cup coconut milk
90 ml coconut oil melted
1/2 cup coconut nectar syrup
2 tbsp freeze dried strawberry powder
1 tbsp nutritional yeast
1 tsp irish moss gel (recipe on the next page)
1 tsp lemon juice
1/4 tsp pink himalayan salt
1/4 cup fresh or frozen raspberries or strawberries

Place the young coconut meat in the blender jar along with the rest of the ingredients (except the strawberry powder, which will be added for the second layer).
Blend until you obtain a smooth, creamy texture, stopping the blender from time to time if needed, to stir the mixture and scrape down the sides of the jar.
Distribute the cream among the parfait glasses. Put 3-4 fresh or defrosted raspberries or strawberries on the white cream.
Add the freeze dried strawberry powder in the other half of the cream. Blend until smooth.
Pour the half of the strawberry cream over the strawberries. Transfer the rest of the cream in a piping bag. Pipe to decorate the jars. Store in the refrigerator at least 4 hours before serving.
Before serving, sprinkle some strawberry powder over the each parfait and garnish with desiccated coconut and edible flowers if desired.

This dessert can be stored in the refrigerator up to 2 days.

HOW TO PREPARE IRISH MOSS GEL

Ingredients

Hydrated irish moss
Filtered water

Thoroughly rinse the dried irish moss under running water to remove all traces of sand and grit.
Let it soak in cold water in the fridge for 3-4 hours, preferably changing the soaking water a couple of times. Use a large container because Irish moss triples in volume while soaking.
Rinse it very well and make sure no traces of sand, dirt or debris from the sea remain.
Add the irish moss to the jar of the blender and blend with a little bit of water until you obtain a smooth gel.
Stop the blender and scrape down the sides of the jar to prevent overheating. Keep adding water until you get the right consistency, but be mindful! Use as little as possible, to maintain the seaweed's gelling power.
Once you obtain a lump-free viscous gel, transfer the mixture to a clean, airtight glass container.

It can be stored in an airtight container
in the fridge for a week or up to 2 months in the freezer.

JUICY CHIA PUDDING

Yield: 2 small bowls

Ingredients

4 tbsp chia seeds
1/2 cup orange juice
1 tbsp finely grated ginger
1/2 cup fresh apple juice
1/2 cup coconut cream
1-2 tsp date syrup
Fresh mint leaves for garnish
Orange zest for garnish

In a medium bowl, gently stir together the chia seeds and the orange juice, apple juice and grated ginger. Cover and set in the refrigerator overnight. Make sure the coconut cream is also set in the refrigerator overnight.

In the morning, give the chia seed pudding a good mix, breaking apart any clumps.

Serve it into individual bowls and set aside.

Beat the coconut cream and sugar together with a hand beater on medium speed for about 3-5 minutes, until light and creamy. Dollop the coconut cream on top of the chia seed pudding.

Gently top the coconut cream with the orange zest and a few mint leaves. Serve immediately.

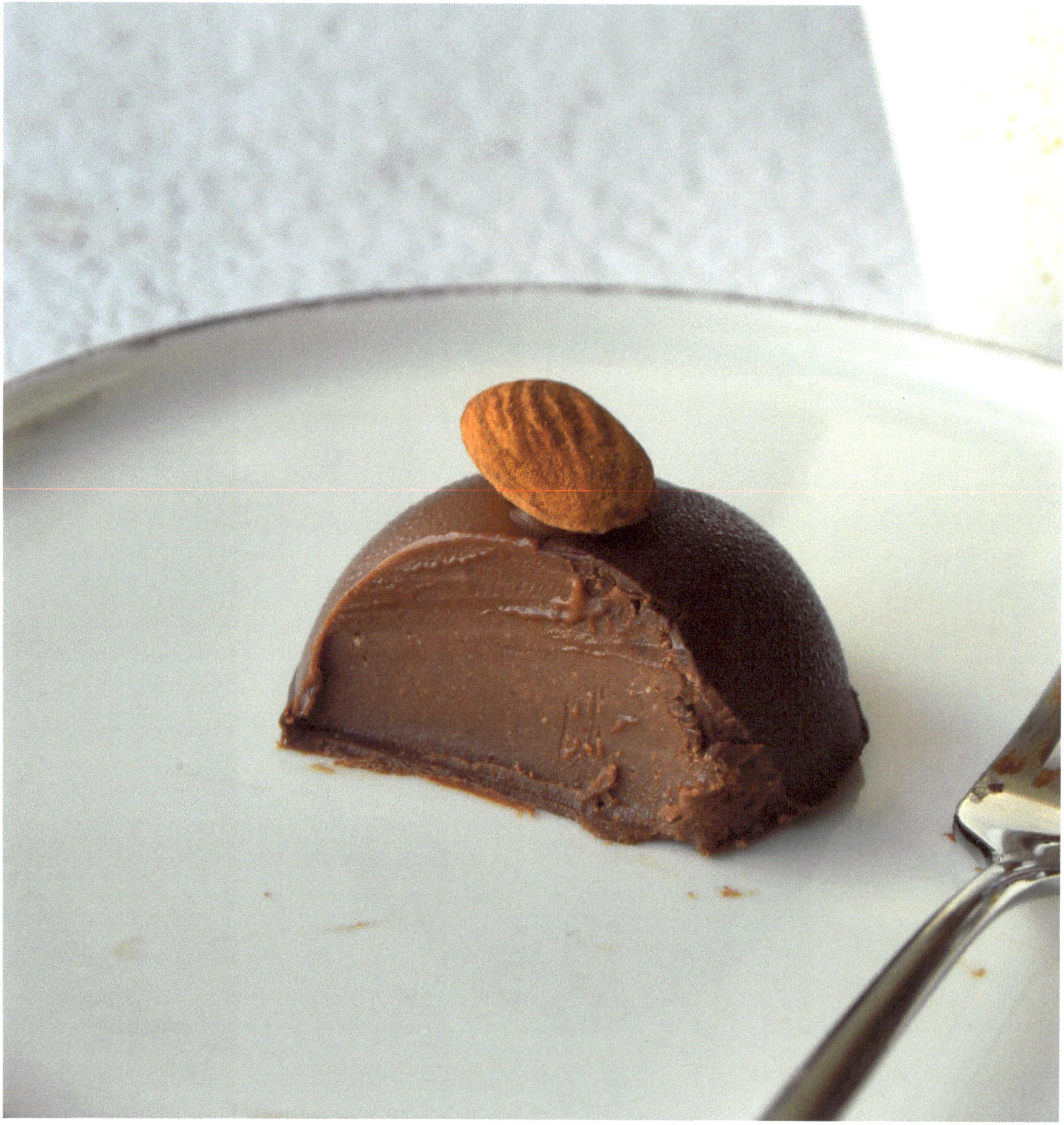

GIANDUJA

Yield: 4

Ingredients

1 cup raw cacao butter melted
1 cup maple syrup
1 cup raw cacao powder
2 vanilla beans scraped
1 tsp medicine flower hazelnut extract
1/2 tsp pink himalayan salt
40 g raw chocolate melted for dipping (optional)
1/4 cup hazelnut or almond for garnish.

Blend the melted raw cacao, vanilla, hazelnut extract and salt together in a high speed blender. I used Blendtec with the Twister Jar.

Then add the maple syrup and raw cacao powder. Blend until completely blended.

Pour the mixture in desired silicon molds.

Store in the refrigerator for 2 hours to set.

Then remove from the refrigerator. Dip the half of the gianduja in melted raw chocolate. Top with hazelnut or almonds for garnish.

Let it sit in the refrigerator for 1 hour before serving.

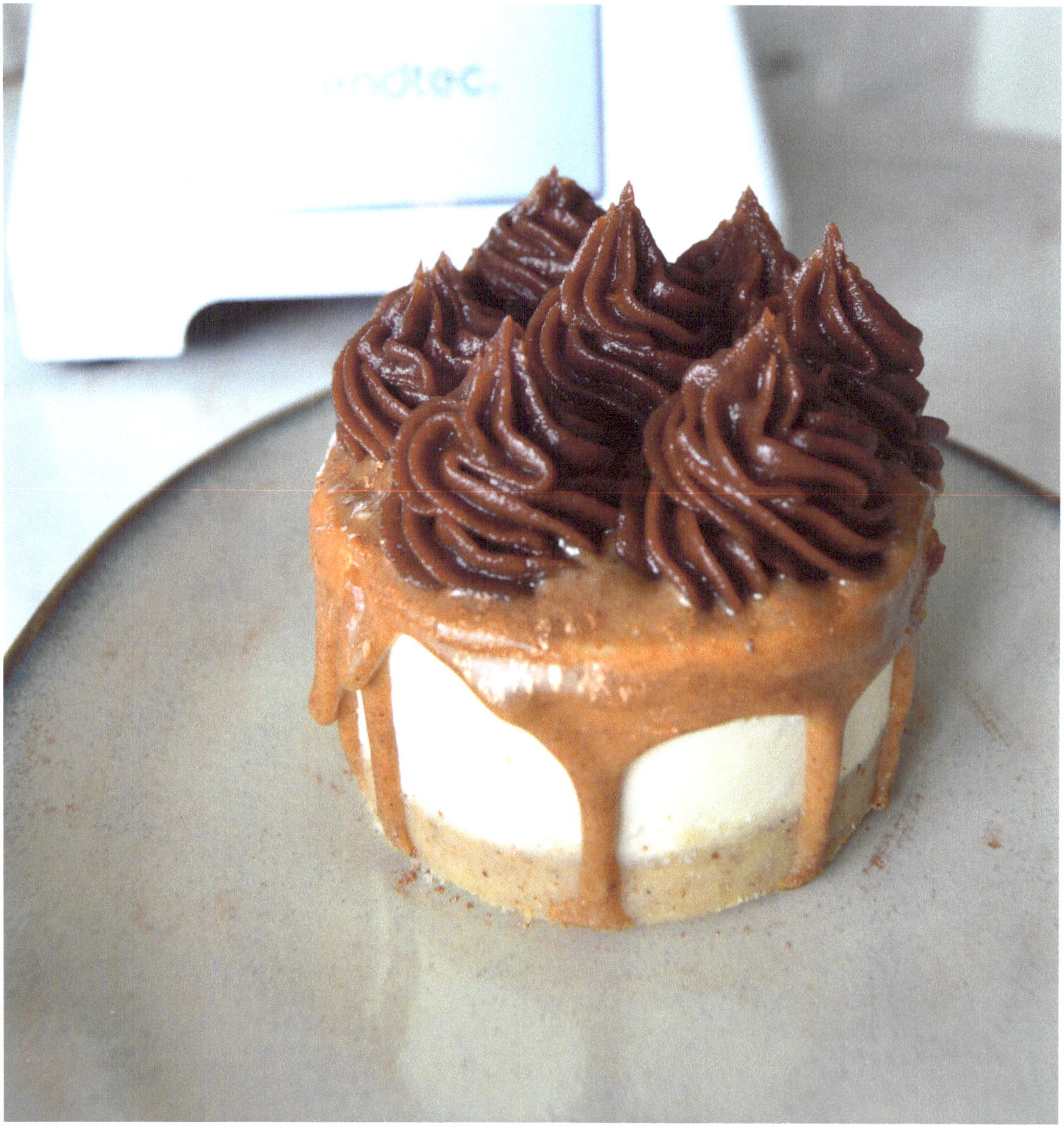

APPLE PECAN CAKE WITH CARAMEL

Yield: 3 x 7 cm round cake

Crust

1 cup pecans
1 cup almonds
1 tbsp almond butter
10 large dates pitted
A pinch of salt

Filling

2 cups cashews soaked
4 red apples peeled, seeds removed
2 tsp maca powder
2 tsp cinnamon powder
1/4 cup coconut oil melted
1/3 cup raw cacao butter melted
1/3 cup maple syrup
3 tbsp lemon juice
1 cup almond milk

Caramel

1/2 to 1 cup water as needed
2 tbsp melted raw cacao butter
10 large soft dates pitted
2 tbsp pecan butter
A pinch of salt

To make filling, soak the cashew nuts in clean water with a pinch of salt for min 4 hours.
Line 7 cm spring form or loose-bottomed cake tine with plastic wrap (it will be easier to remove the bottom part of the tin from the cake).
To make the crust, in a food processor, first, process nuts until small crumbles, and then add dates, pecan butter and salt. Blitz to combine and process until well incorporated and mixture starts to stick together. Turn out into the prepared tin and press down to form an even base. Freeze.
To make filling, rinse and drain cashew nuts thoroughly and add it to the blender along with the rest of the ingredients. Process until you get very smooth and creamy batter.
Pour the mix over the prepared crust. Put into the freezer for min for 4 hours or until set.
When set, decorate with caramel and , if you wish, pipe avocado frosting on top (you'll find the recipe in this book)
Decorate with figs or dried apple chips if you like.
To make caramel, process dates, water and sea salt in the blender until smooth and a little bit runny. Start with ¼ cup of water and gradually add more until you reach desired consistency. Lastly add the melted cacao butter and blend well. Recipe makes about 1 cup of caramel, store any leftovers in the fridge for up to 5 days.
Store cake in the freezer, but let it stand outside for about 1 hour or so before serving.

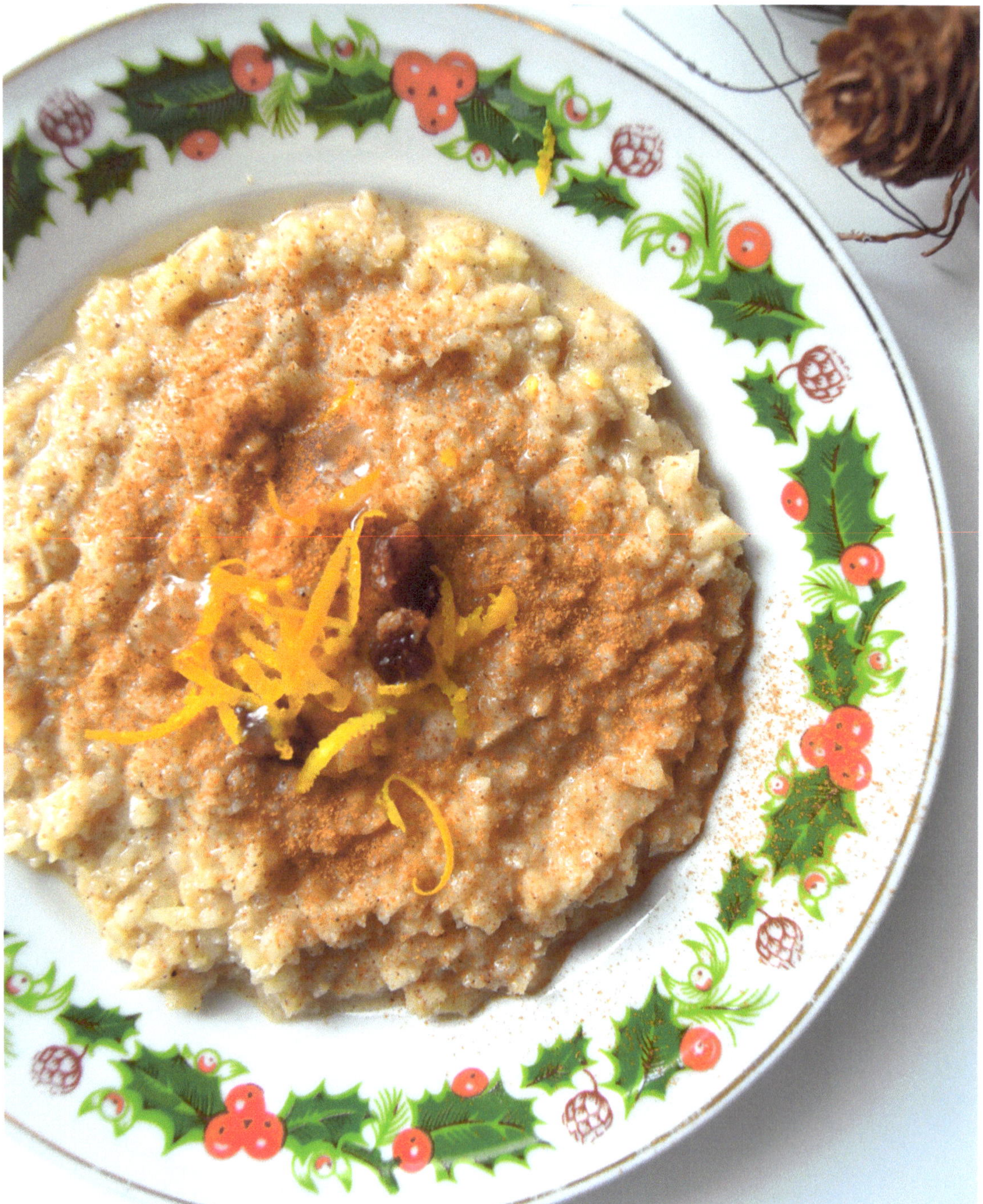

TOMTEGRÖT - CHRISTMAS PORRIDGE

Yield: 2 person

Ingredients

1 small swede(a.k.a rutabaga) OR kohlrabi (135g)
50 g almonds blanced, soaked for 30 minutes or almond butter
80 ml fresh orange juice (juice of 1 whole orange)
1 tsp coconut oil (optional, check the last step)
1 tbsp maple syrup
1/8 tsp ground cardamom
1 tsp cinnamon powder
1/2 tsp vanilla bean powder
1/4 tsp ground ginger or grated fresh ginger
A pinch of salt

Peel the swede (rutabaga) or kohlrabi and cut it into chunks around 1" wide.
Blend the swede or kohlrabi pieces in a food processor until they break down to look rice-like.
Transfer them to a nut milk bag in a bowl and squeeze out any excess liquid, alternatively you can use vegan milker.
Discard the liquid and put the rice in a clean bowl.
Blend up the almonds, orange juice, maple, cinnamon, cardamom, vanilla, ginger and a pinch of salt in a high-speed blender until smooth. Add to the swede. Combine well.
Transfer mixture in a large bowl.

OPTIONAL STEP if you want to eat it warm : Cover the bowl with a cling film. Dehydrate at 42-46°C in the Excalibur dehydrator for 30-40 minutes or until warm. Pour 1 tsp coconut oil in the middle of the bowl and let it melt for 2-3 minutes. Finely peel the orange, put orange zest on your bowl, along with the raisins. Dust some cinnamon powder if desired. Enjoy.

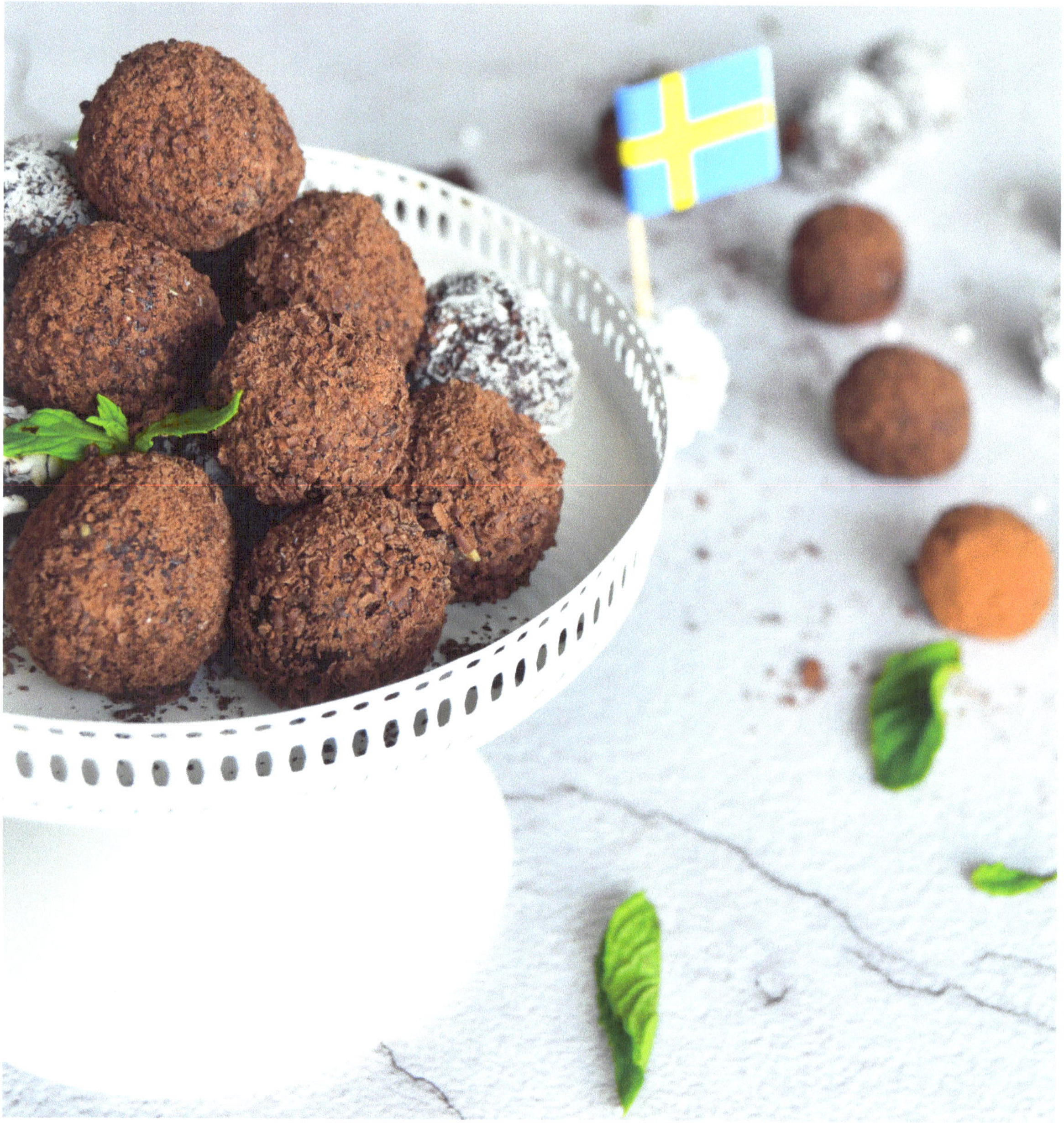

SWEDISH CHOCOLATE BALLS

Yield: 10-12 balls

Ingredients

100 g sprouted rolled oats
50 g activated dehydrated almonds
100 g soft medjool dates
2 tbsp raw cacao powder
2 tbsp carob powder
1 tsp vanilla bean powder
2 tbsp maple syrup
2-3 tbsp cold press espresso
1/4 tsp salt
1/4 cup desiccated coconut and shredded raw chocolate to decorate

Place the oats, almonds, cacao powder, carob powder, vanilla bean powder and salt in the food processor. Blend until everything combined well and you get a flour-like mixture. Then add the medjool dates, maple and espresso. Blend until you get a sticky dough. Taste it if you need add more maple or salt.

Make smal balls with your hands.

Roll the balls in desiccated coconut or shredded raw chocolate.

Place in an airtight container, set in the refrigerator at least 1-2 hours before serving.

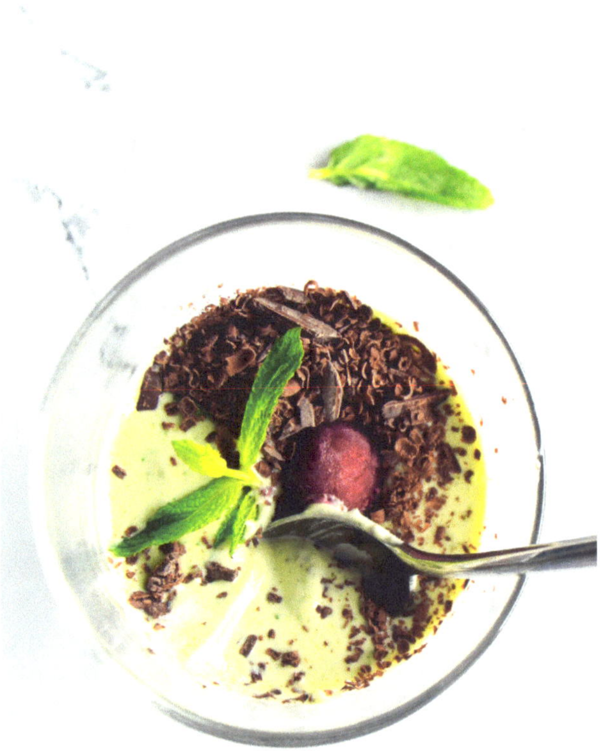

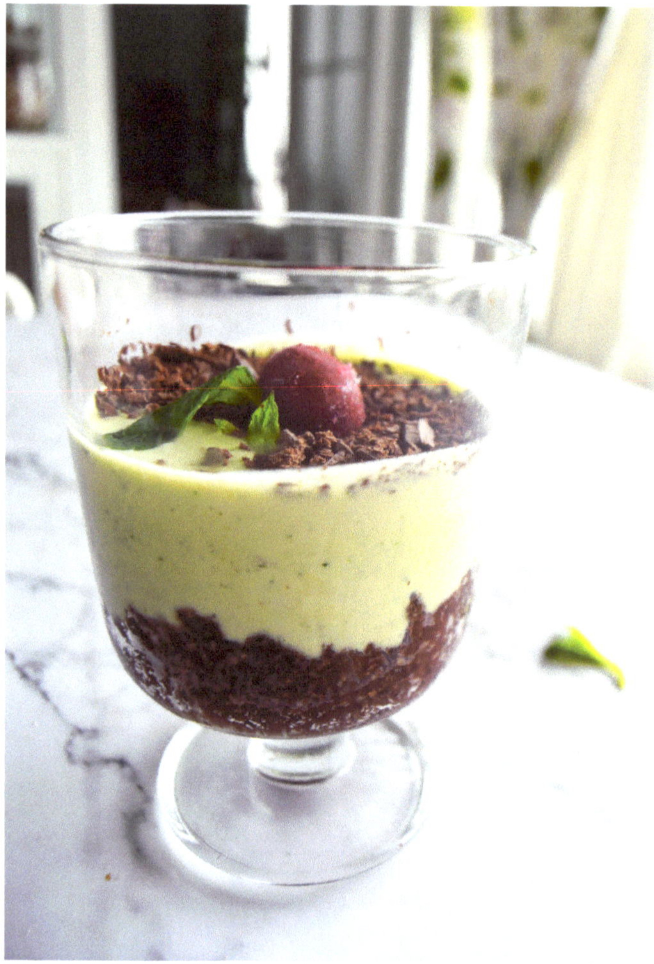

PEPPERMINT CHOCOLATE PARFAITS

Yield: 3-4 person

Crust

1 cup hazelnut meal
4-5 large medjool dates pitted
2 tbsp raw cacao powder
1 tsp vanilla bean powder
A pinch licorice salt

Cream

2 cups raw cashews
1/4 cup fresh mint
1/2 cup coconut milk
4 tbsp lemon juice
2 tbsp maple syrup
2-3 drops mint essential oil
1 tbsp coconut oil
1/4 tsp ground cardamom

Toppings

Cherries
Shredded raw chocolate
Fresh mint leaves

Place all the crust ingredients into the food processor. Mix on high speed until you get sticky dough. Spread out evenly into little parfait jar. Keep in the refrigerator while you are making the cream.

Place all the filling ingredients into your blender, mix on very high speed until you get silky smooth mixture. Taste it. If you like intense flavour, add more little bit more mint essential oil.

Remove the jars from the refrigerator. Pour the mixture over the crust. Put in the refrigerator for 2 hours before serving.

Then decorate with cherry or your favorite fruit, mint leaves and shredded chocolate. Serve cold!

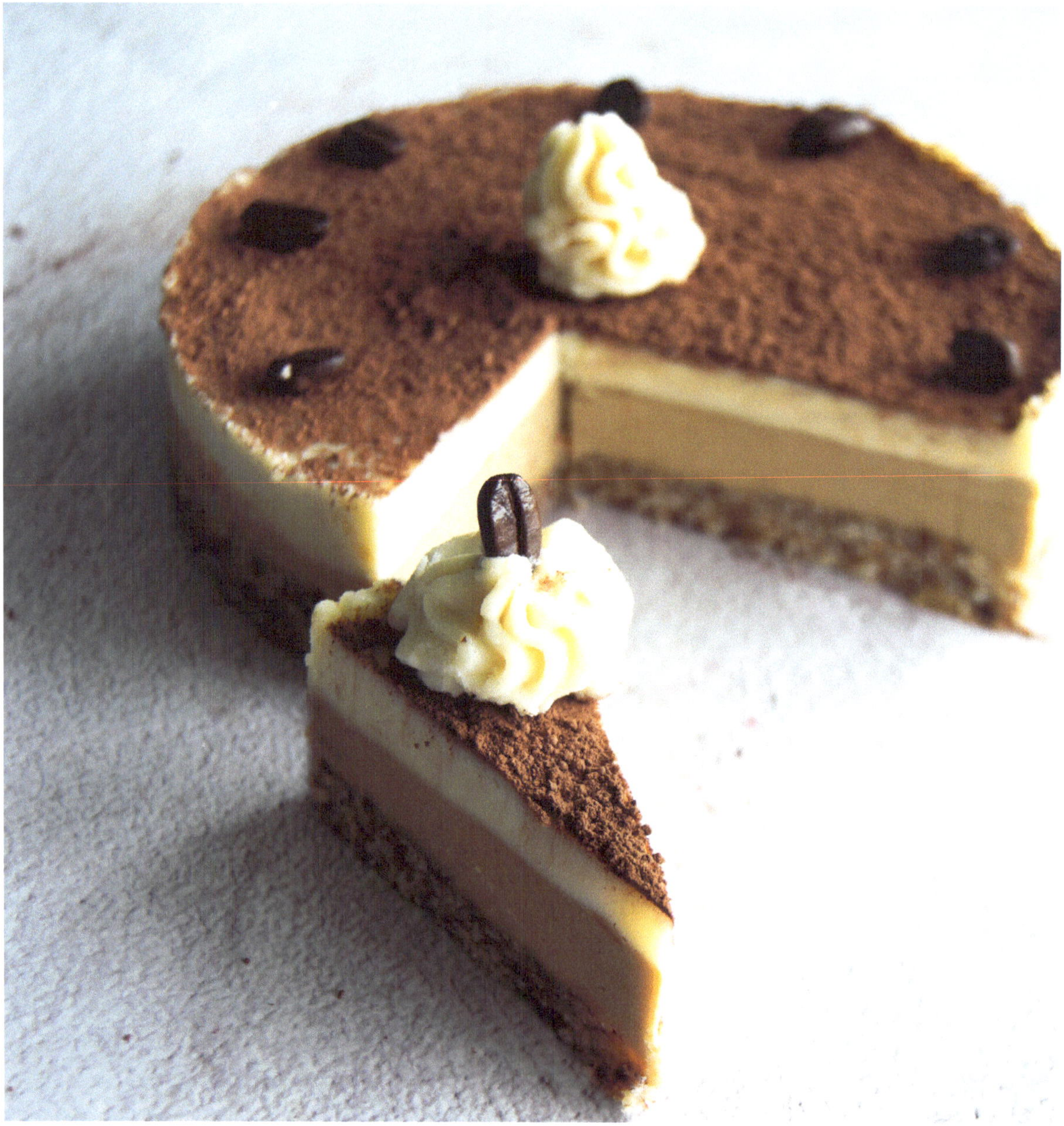

TIRAMISU CAKE

Yield: 16 cm round cake

Crust

1/2 cup hazelnut flour
1/2 cup tigernut flour
1/2 cup medjool dates pitted
2 tbsp hazelnut butter
1/4 tsp salt

Coffee Layer

1 cup raw cashews soaked
1 tbsp raw cacao butter melted
2 tbsp maple syrup
3 tbsp cold press espresso
1 tbsp coconut oil melted
1 tbsp raw cacao powder
3-4 tbsp cashew milk as needed to blend
1 tsp vanilla bean powder

White Cream Layer

1 cup young coconut meat
40 g raw cacao butter melted
2 tbsp maple syrup
1 tbsp coconut oil
1 tsp lemon juice
1/4 cup coconut milk as needed to blend

Process all crust layer ingredients in your food processor until you get a sticky dough. Press the mixture into cake tin, press down well and place in the freezer to set while you work with your filling.

Place the soaked strained cashews in the Blendtec Twister Jar. Add the cashew milk, espresso and maple syrup. Blend well until smooth. Then add the vanilla bean powder, raw cacao powder, melted cacao butter and coconut oil. Blend well until everything combined well and you get a silky smooth mixture.

Pour the coffee layer over the crust. Freeze while you are making the white cream.

Place the young coconut meat in the Blendtec Twister Jar. Add the coconut milk, lemon juice and maple , then blend until smooth cream. Then add the melted raw cacao butter and coconut oil. Blend until silky smooth.

Set 2 tbsp of the white cream layer aside to decorate later if you wish.

Pour the rest of the white cream over the coffee layer.

Dust some raw cacao powder on top if you like.

Pipe the remaining 2 tbsp of the white cream on the cake.

Drop some coffee beans on the top of cake.

Store in the refrigerator for 4 hours before serving.

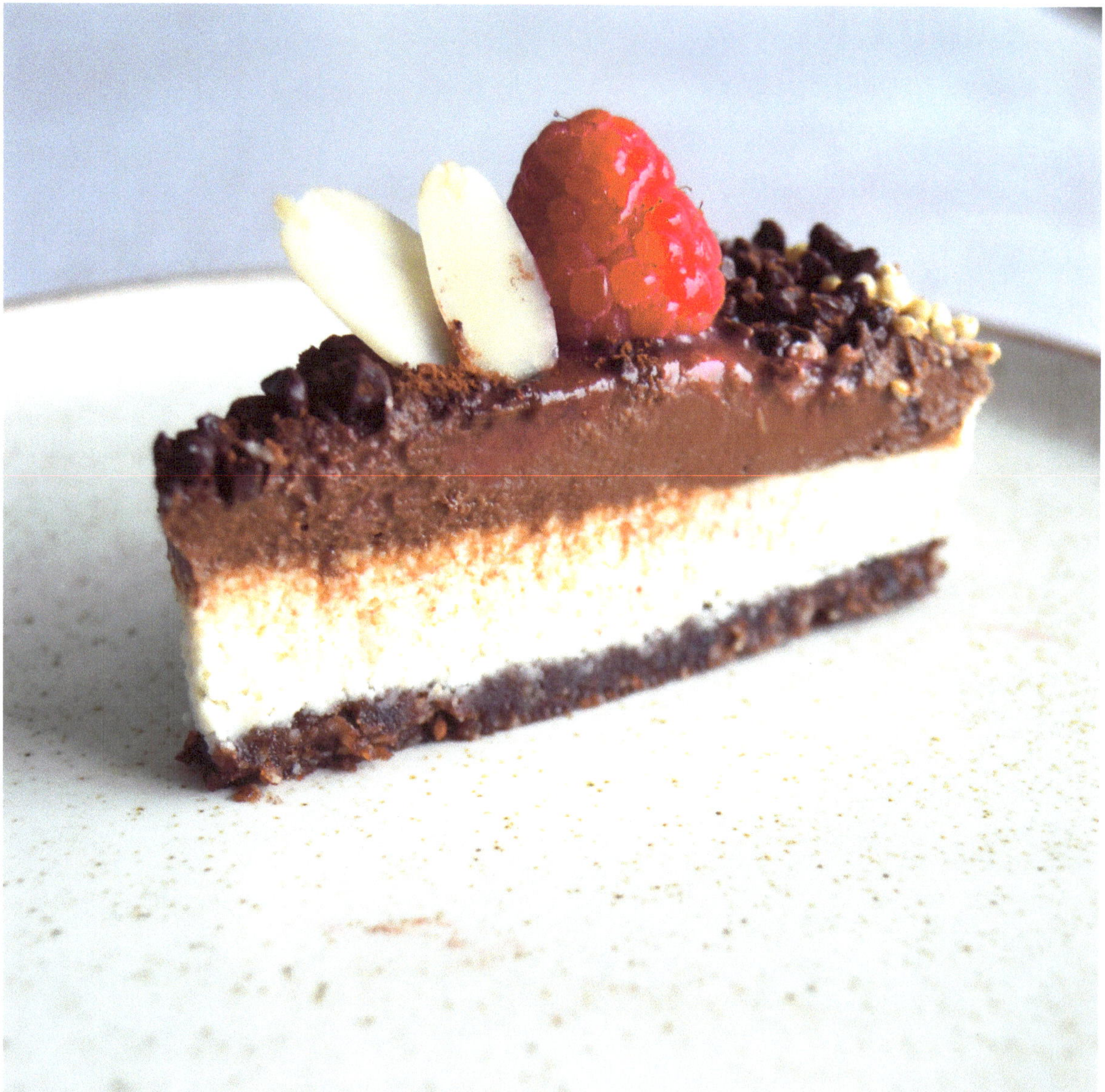

OUR SIGNATURE CAKE

Yield: 16 cm round cake

Crust

160 g almond meal
160 g soft medjool dates pitted
2 tbsp coconut oil or almond butter
1 tbsp raw cacao powder
1/4 tsp pink himalayan salt

Middle Layer

130 g cashews soaked
100 g coconut cream (only fatty part)
2 tbsp maple syrup
3 tbsp lemon juice
2 tbsp coconut oil melted
1 tbsp raw cacao butter melted
1 tsp vanilla bean powder

Chocolate Layer

250 g ripe avocado (weight after peeled and core removed)
2 tbsp lemon juice
1 tbsp raw cacao powder
1 tbsp maple syrup
180 g raw dark chocolate melted

Place all crust ingredients into the food processor, mix on high speed until you get dough. Line a parchment paper into the spring-form pan (16 cm) Transfer dough to the spring-form pan. Press using the back of spoon, flatten out.
Place all the middle layer ingredients except raw cacao butter and coconut oil into the blender mix on high speed until get silky and smooth mixture. Lastly add the coconur oil and raw cacao butter. Blend until well combined.
Pour mixture onto the crust layer, flatten out using a spatula. Place it to the freezer while preparing chocolate layer.
Place the avocados, lemon juice, maple and raw cacao powder into the food processor, mix on high speed until smooth. Using a double boiler, melt raw chocolate slowly maximum at 42 degrees. Then add to the food processor, mix with the avocado mixture on high speed until get silky smooth texture.
Pour mixture onto the white layer.
Garnish with almond slices, fresh, raspberries, edible flowers and raw cacao nibs if desired. Let it cool in refrigerator at least 4 hours before serving.

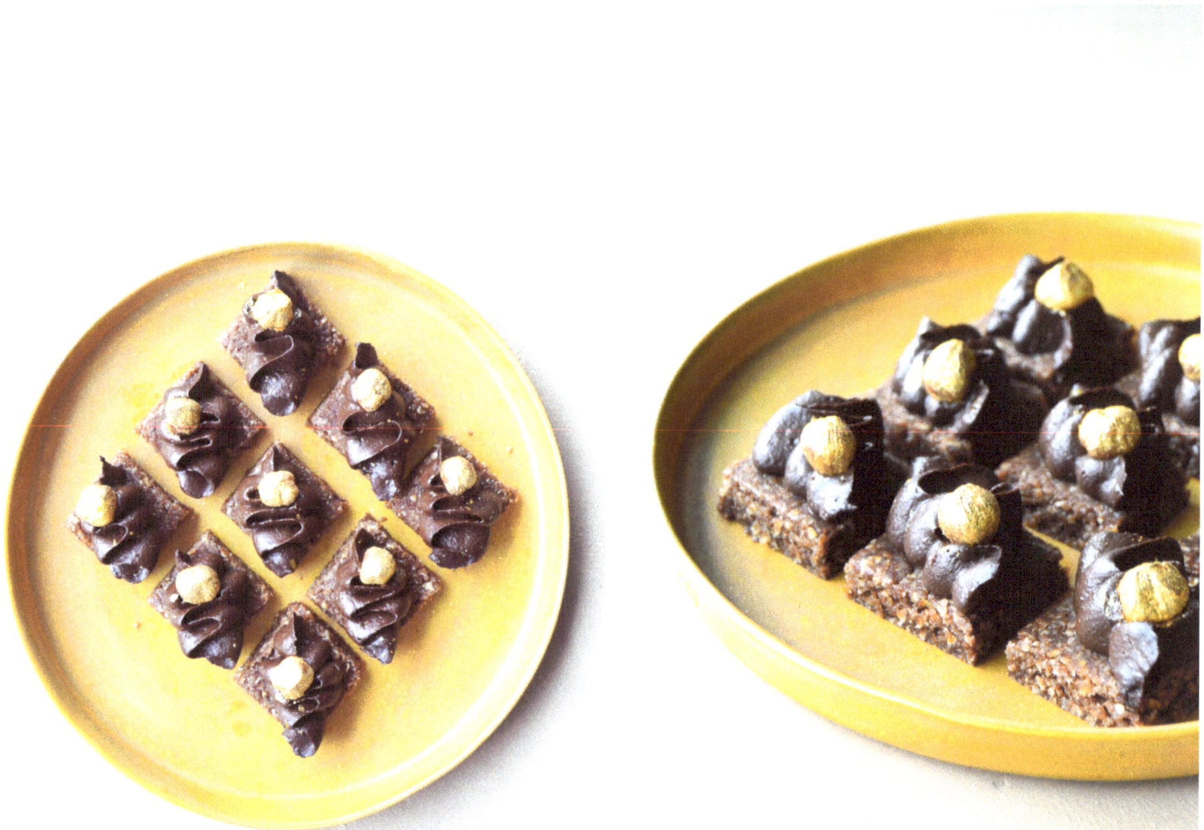

RAW BLONDIES WITH AVOCADO CHOCOLATE FROSTING

Yield: 8-10 balls

Ingredients

90 g gluten free rolled oats
140 g smooth hazelnut butter
1/4 tsp pink himalayan salt
1 tsp vanilla bean powder
1 tsp raw cacao
3-4 tbsp hazelnut milk
1/2 cup hazelnuts to decorate

Avocado Frosting

1 perfectly ripe avocado
1 tbsp raw cacao powder
30 g melted raw chocolate
3-4 tbsp maple syrup
A pinch salt
1/4 vanilla bean powder

Place rolled oats, salt, vanilla and cacao in the food processor, blend to combine.
Then add the hazelnut butter and milk. Process until you get dough.
Transfer mixture in a 20x20 cm baking tin lined parchment paper. Press down the dough. Using a spatula, flatten out. Set in the refrigerator. while you are making the frosting.
To make avocado frosting, halve and pit the avocados, then scoop them into a food processor fitted with a steel blade or high-powered blender.
Add the raw cacao powder, maple, melted chocolate, vanilla extract, and salt. Blend until very smooth and creamy, stopping to scrape down the bowl as needed.
Taste and add a few teaspoons of maple if additional sweetness is desired.
Transfer frosting in a pipping bag with wilton petal piping tip no 125, let it cool in the refrigerator for about 10 minutes. 8. Meanwhile, cut your brownies in small squares. Then decorate your brownies with the frosting. Top with hazelnuts.

Notes: If you don't have piping tip, just by using a spatula, spread the frosting over the blondies. Recipe is also delicious without the frosting, can be made naked.

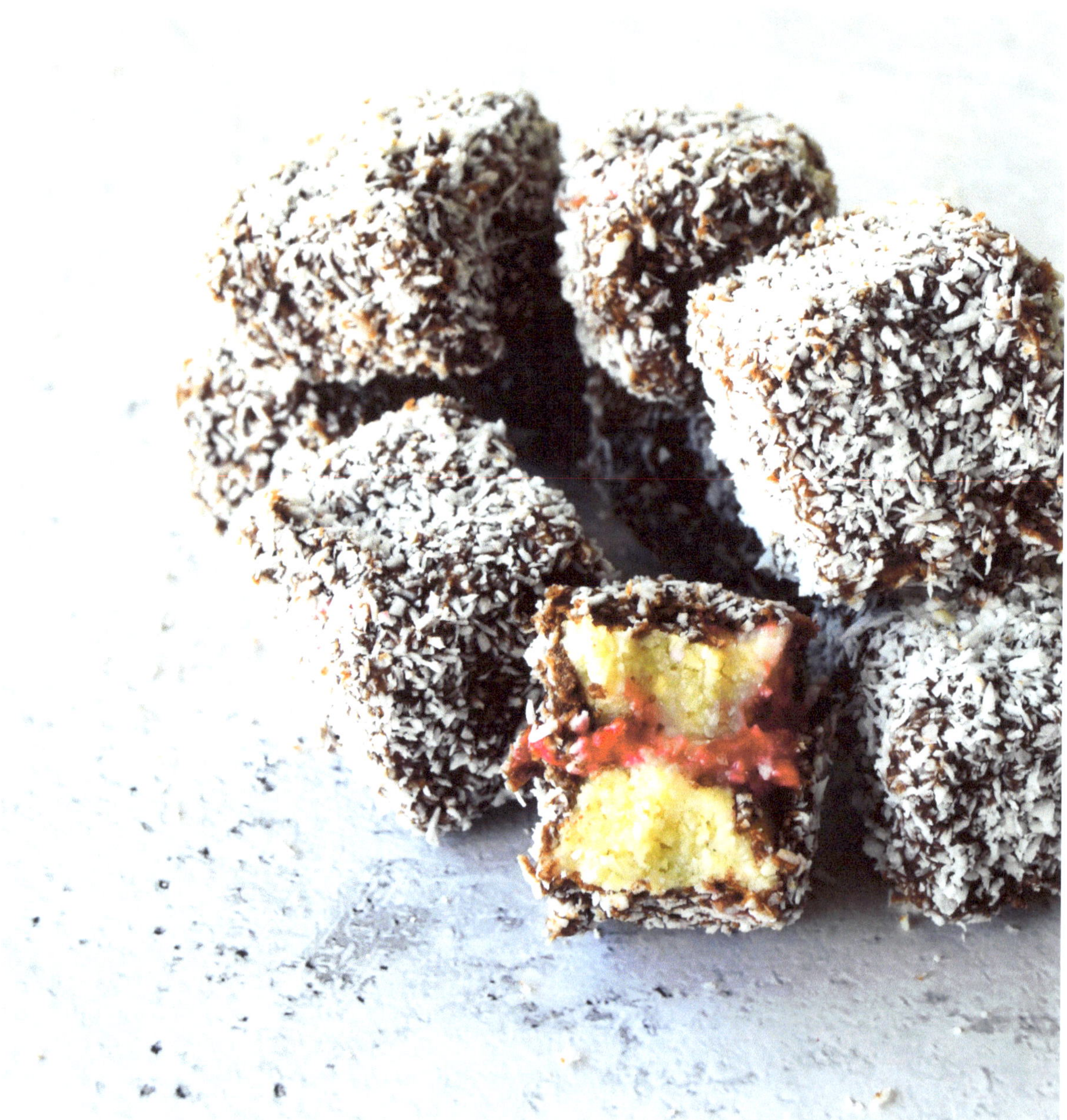

COCONUT RASPBERRY LAMINGTONS

Yield: 14-16 lamingtons

Sponge

3 cups raw cashews

1 + 1/2 cups desiccated coconut

1/2 cup coconut cream (only fatty part)

1/2 cup maple syrup

Raspberry Chia Jam

1 + 1/2 cups raspberries

2 tbsp chia seeds

1 tbsp maple syrup

Coconut Cream

1 + 1/2 cup young coconut meat

1/2 cup coconut cream (only fatty part)

2 tbsp coconut oil

1 tbsp maple syrup

Coating

1/2 cup raw cacao butter melted

1/4 cup coconut cream (only fatty part)

1/4 tbsp raw cacao powder

2 tbsp maple syrup

2 cups desiccated coconut

Line two pyrex with parchment papers.

To prepare the sponge, add the cashews to a food processor and process until it forms fine crumbs. Add the remaining ingredients to the food processor and pulse until just combined. Do not over process the mixture otherwise you'll end up with a very solid sponge. We want it soft.

Halve the sponge mixture and press each mixture into your lined containers. Set aside in the fridge.

To make the raspberry chia jam, mash the raspberries with a fork and mix through the chia seeds and optional sweetener. Set aside to thicken while making the cream.

To make the coconut cream, add all ingredients to a high-speed blender and blend until it forms a very smooth cream. Remove and set it aside in fridge.

To make the coating, melt all ingredients except the desiccated coconut over a double boiler. Mix until well combined.

To assemble, remove the chilled sponge'from the pyrexs. 8. Place one sponge on top of the other and cut into even-sized pieces.

Using a fork, dip a sponge into the chocolate (dip all sides except one) then quickly dip into the coconut and set aside. Repeat for the remaining sponge cakes.

Separate the iced sponge cakes into 2 groups. Spread raspberry chia jam on the plain side of one group of sponge cakes. Spread coconut cream on the plain side of the other half of sponge cakes. Sandwich together a sponge with jam and a sponge with cream.

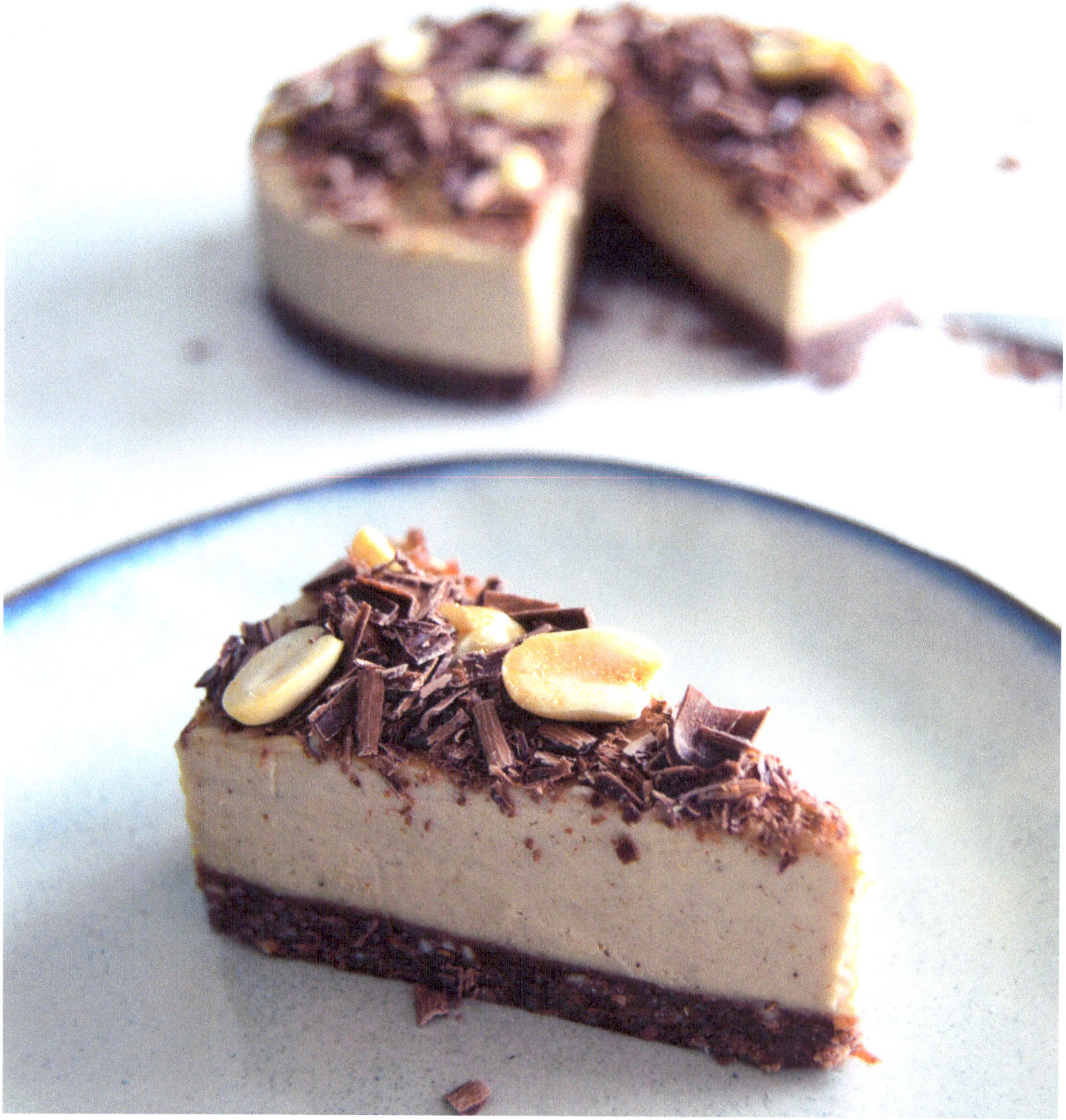

PEANUT BANANA CAKE

Yield: 15 cm round cake

Crust
1/2 cup peanuts
1/2 cup almond flour
1/2 cup buckinis
3 tbsp raw cacao powder
3 tbsp maple syrup
2 tbsp coconut oil
1/2 tsp salt

Cream
4 frozen bananas
1/2 cup peanut butter
1/4 cup maple syrup
2 tbsp coconut oil
1 tsp vanilla bean powder
1/2 tsp salt
1/2 tsp cinnamon powder

Toppings
Peanuts and chocolate shavings

Process all crust ingredients in a food processor until the mixture is combined and starts to form into a ball. Transfer to a 15 cm springform pan and press down into a flat even crust along the bottom. Freeze while working on next step.

Wipe out the processor to remove any remaining residues from the crust. Add all filling ingredients to the processor and process into a smooth creamy texture.

Transfer this mixture into the springform pan over the crust. Tap the pan on the counter a few times (to release air bubbles) and smooth out the top of the cake with the back of a spoon. Decorate with peanuts and chocolate shavings toppings.

Freeze for 6 hours or overnight to set. Remove from pan, slice and serve. Keep leftovers frozen.

COCONUT CHIA PUDDING

Yield: 2 small bowls

Ingredients

60 g chia seeds
1 tbsp lime zest
1 tbsp lime juice
200 ml coconut milk
200 ml coconut water
Fresh strawberries to serve
Coconut chips to serve

Combine the chia seeds, lime zest, coconut milk and coconut water in a small bowl. Cover and refrigerate for at least 1–2 hours or overnight, stirring occasionally, until thickened. If the pudding becomes too thick, thin with a little water, coconut milk or coconut water to the consistency you like.

Taste the pudding and add a squeeze of lime juice to balance the flavour to your liking.

Serve the chia pudding into bowls and top with strawberries, coconut chips and lime zest.

RASPBERRY BEETROOT SMOOTHIE

Yield: 2 small bowls

Ingredients

1/2 cup fresh apple juice
1/2 cup cashew milk
1/2 cup fresh beetroot juice
1 cup fresh raspberries
1/2 cup raw cacao powder
2 tbsp maca powder
2 ripe avocados peeled and core removed
1 tsp vanilla bean powder
1 tbsp coconut nectar syrup or more as needed

Add the avocados, apples and beet juice into your blender. Mix on high speed until smooth.

Then add all remaining ingredients and mix well together. Transfer the mixture to a bowl, cover, and chill in the fridge for 2-3 hours to thicken. Serve topped with fresh raspberries if desired.

COCONUT LEMON MACAROONS

Yield: 10-12 macaroons

Ingredients

2 cups raw cashews
6 cups shredded coconut
3 tbsp lemon zest
1 tbsp coconut oil melted
1/2 cup maple syrup
1/2 cup lemon juice
2 tsp vanilla bean powder
1/2 tsp cardamom powder

Soak cashews overnight, wash, drain and dehydrate until fully dried. Then throw the cashews into a food processor and pulse until ground into a fine flour.

Add the shredded coconut, lemon zest, and cardamom, and pulse a few times until well combined. Add the lemon juice, maple syrup, coconut oil, and vanilla, then pulse until well combined. Transfer the mixture to a large bowl, and using a tablespoon, scoop out balls, and with your hands shape them into mounds.

Place the macaroons on mesh dehydrator sheets, and sprinkle more cardamom if you like. Dehydrate in your dehydrator at 42 degrees for 8 to 12 hours, or until texture is achieved

HAZELNUT TRUFFLES

Yield: 6-8 balls

Ingredients

75 g hazelnut butter
4 tbsp raw cacao butter melted
4 tbsp raw cacao powder
3 tbsp maple syrup
2 tbsp hazelnut milk
1/2 tsp vanilla bean powder

Blend the hazelnut butter, hazelnut milk, maple syrup, vanilla extract, in a high speed blender until you get smooth paste.

Add the melted cacao butter and add cacao powder at last. Don't overblend.

Pour the batter into a bowl and refrigerate until firm, it takes about 2 hours.

Roll the mixture into 1-2,5 cm balls. If the dough is too soft and sticky place it again in the refrigerator for a few minutes.

Roll each ball into the topping of your choice. Cacao nibs, coconut flakes or cacao powder are good choices. Store in the refrigerator up to 2-3 weeks.

TIPS
Make sure all the ingredients are at room temperature before starting.

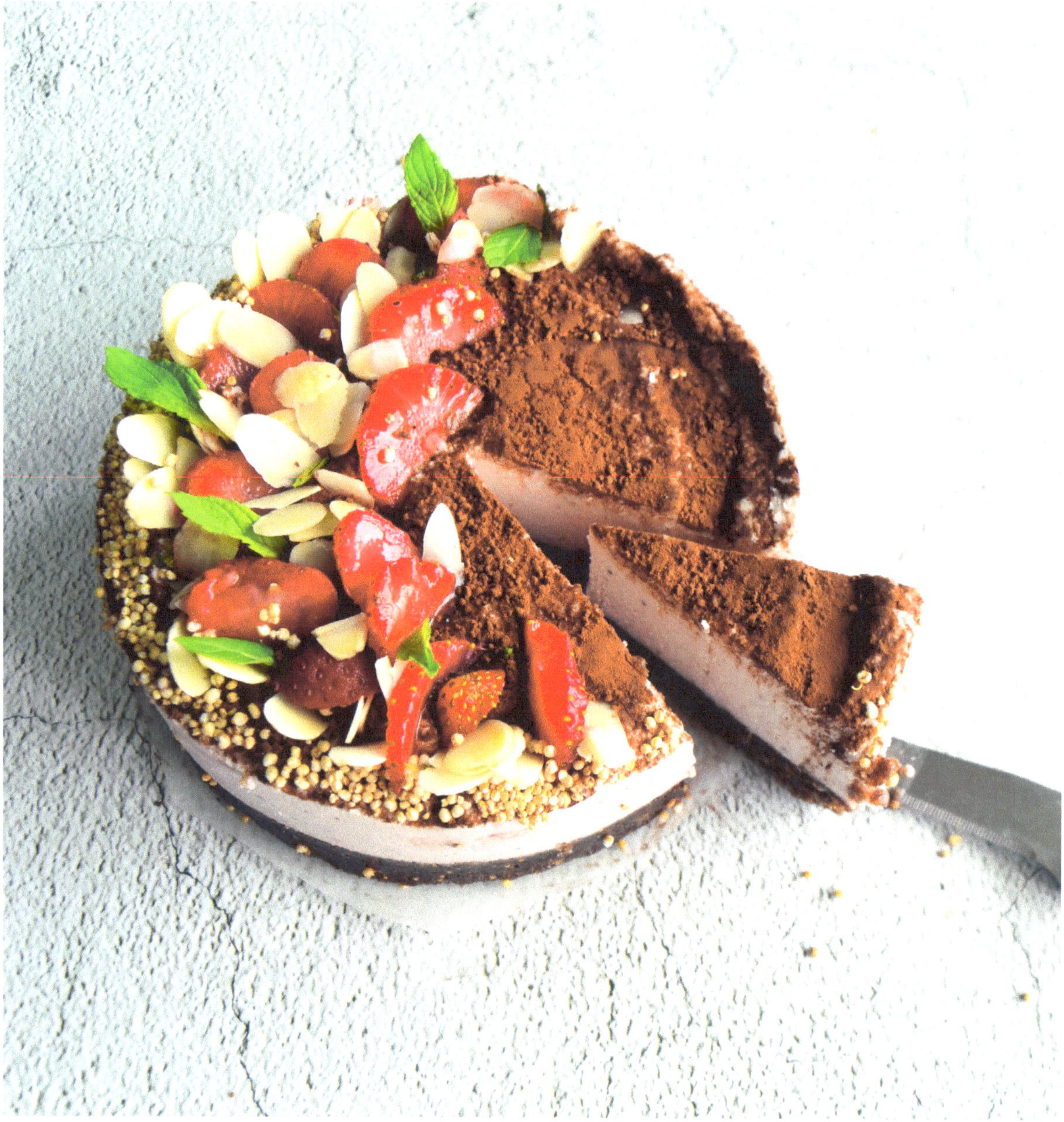

STRAWBERRY CHEESECAKE

Yield: 15 cm round cake

Crust

1/2 cup raw almonds
6 soft medjool dates, pitted and chopped
1 tsp almond butter
1/2 tsp vanilla bean powder
Pinch of salt

Filling

1 + 1/2 cup cashews soaked
1/2 cup cashew milk
1/4 cup lemon juice
3 tbsp coconut oil melted
1 tsp lemon zest
2 tbsp maple syrup
1 tsp nutritional yeast
1/2 tsp vanilla bean powder
1/4 tsp salt
1/2 cup fresh strawberries + more for garnish
Fresh mint leaves for garnish
Sliced almonds for garnish

In a food processor pulse the almonds until partially broken.

Add the chopped dates, vanilla, almond butter, and salt and process until a sticky dough is formed.
Press into a 15 cm spring mold and form.
Place into the freezer for 30 min until it firms up.

To prepare the filling, first rinse and drain the cashews.

Blend all ingredients together (except coconut oil) in a high-speed blender until nice and smooth.

Add the coconut oil and blend again at slow speed just for a few seconds until well incorporated.

Pour the cream over the crust

Place the cake into the freezer for at least 3 hours.

One hour before serving, remove the cheesecake from the mold and place into the refrigerator.

Garnish the top of the cake with strawberries, almond slices and mint.

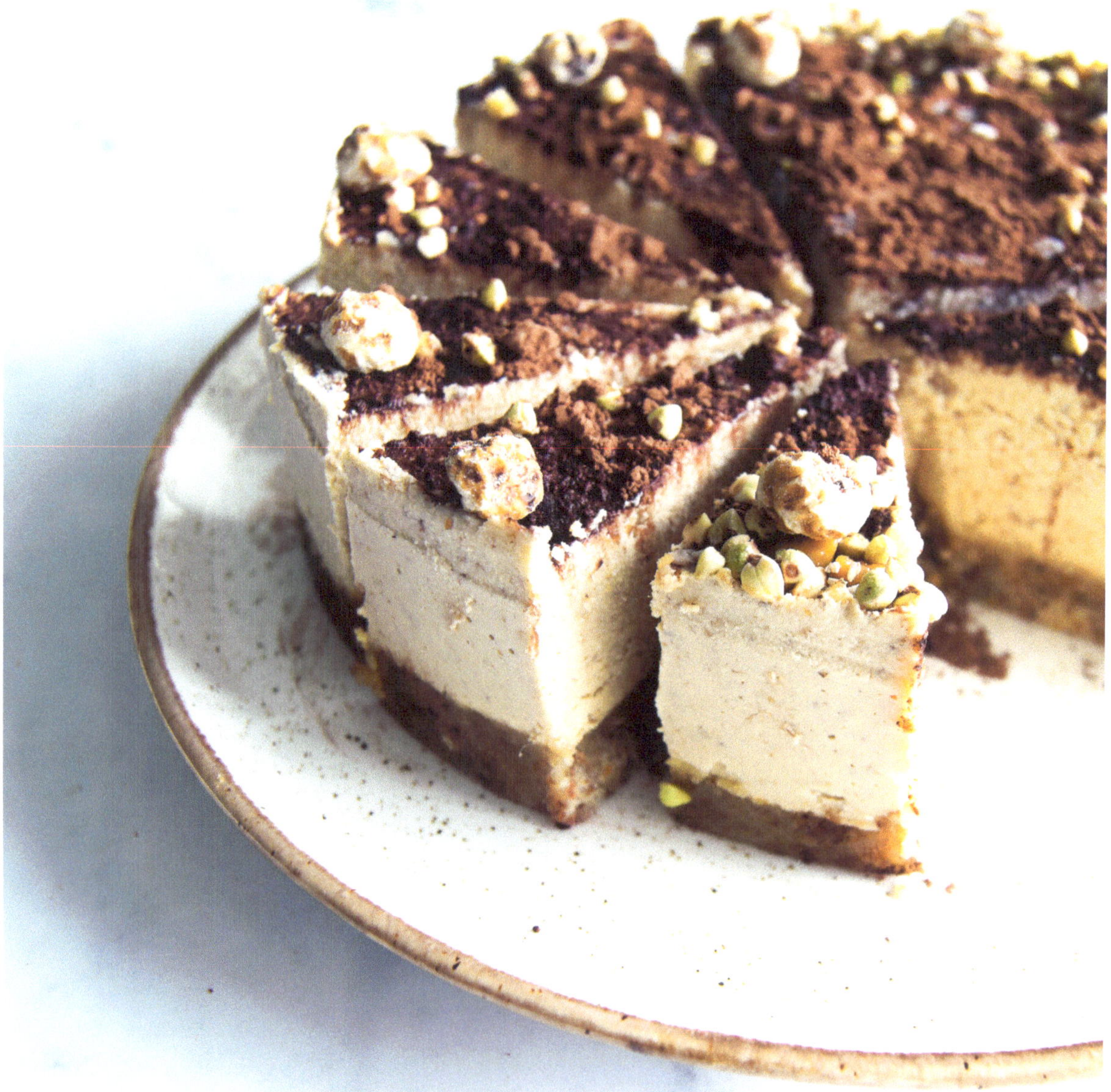

TIGERNUT CHEESECAKE

Yield: 15 cm round cake

Crust

50 g tigernut flour
45 g buckinis
1 tbsp coconut oil melted
110 g soft medjool dates pitted
1/4 tsp pink himalayan salt

Filling

150 g tigernuts soaked
4 tbsp coconut oil melted
5 tbsp maple syrup
3 tbsp lemon juice
1 tsp vanilla bean powder
1/4 tsp licorice salt

Process all crust ingredients in a food processor until a dough mixture forms. Transfer this mixture into a spring form pan and press down into an even crust along the base. Place in the freezer while working on the next step.

Process all filling ingredients (except coconut oil) in a high speed blender until completely smooth. Then add the melted coconut oil, and continue to blend until silky smooth.

Pour mixture over the crust.

Refrigerate at least 4-5 hours before removing from the pan and serving.

Garnish with buckinis and tigernuts. Dust some raw cacao powder on top if desired.

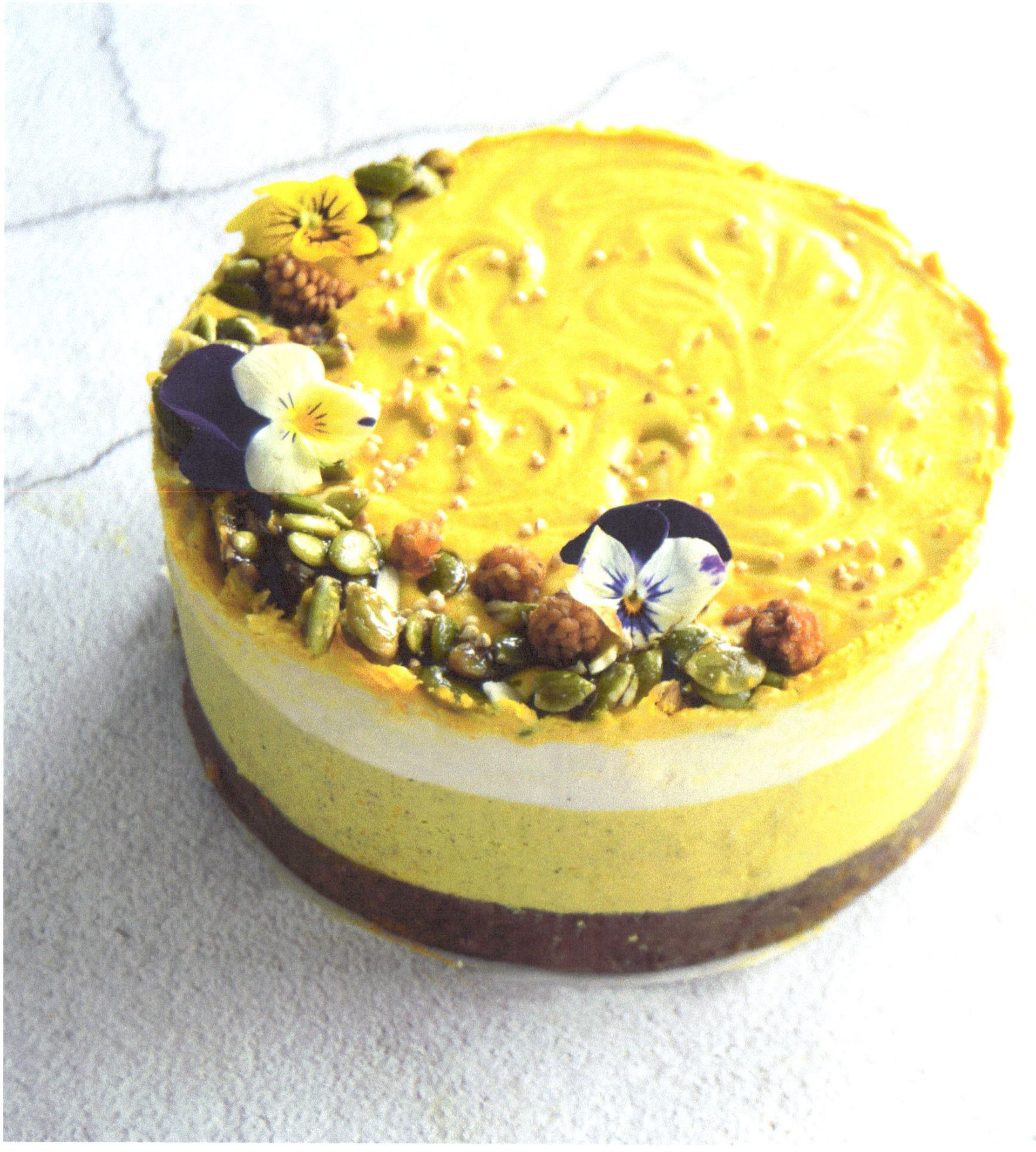

SUNSHINE CHEESECAKE

Yield: 15 cm round cake

Crust

150 g almond meal
4 large soft medjool dates pitted
2 tbsp mulberry powder
1 tbsp almond butter
1-2 tbsp plant milk as needed
A pinch of salt

White Filling

100 g coconut cream
130 g raw cashews soaked
2 tbsp maple syrup
2 tbsp coconut oil
1 tsp vanilla bean powder
2 tbsp lemon juice

Yellow Filling

100 g raw cashews soaked
140 g coconut cream
3 tbsp lemon juice
2 tbsp maple syrup
3 tbsp coconut oil
2 tsp turmeric powder
1 tbsp cinnamon powder
1/2 tsp cardamom powder
1/4 tsp nutmeg powder
2 tsp grounc ginger powder

Process all crust layer ingredients in your food processor until sticky. Press the mixture into cake tin and place in the freezer to set while you work with your filling.

In a food processor, process all yellow cream layer ingredients except coconut oil until smooth. Then add the coconut oil, blend again. Once done, set aside 1/4 of the mixture to use later and spread the rest of the yellow mixture evenly over the base layer, return the cake to the freezer.

Place all the white filling ingredients to the blender except coconut oil. Blend until well combined and creamy. Then add the melted coconut oil, blend until silky smooth. After 30 minutes, remove the cake from the freezer, pour the mixture over the yellow layer.Freeze for another 30 minutes.

Once done, lastly pour the remaining 1/4 of the yellow cream over the white layer.
Decorate with dried mulberries candided peptias and edible flowers if desired. (Check the next page to see how to make candided pepitas)

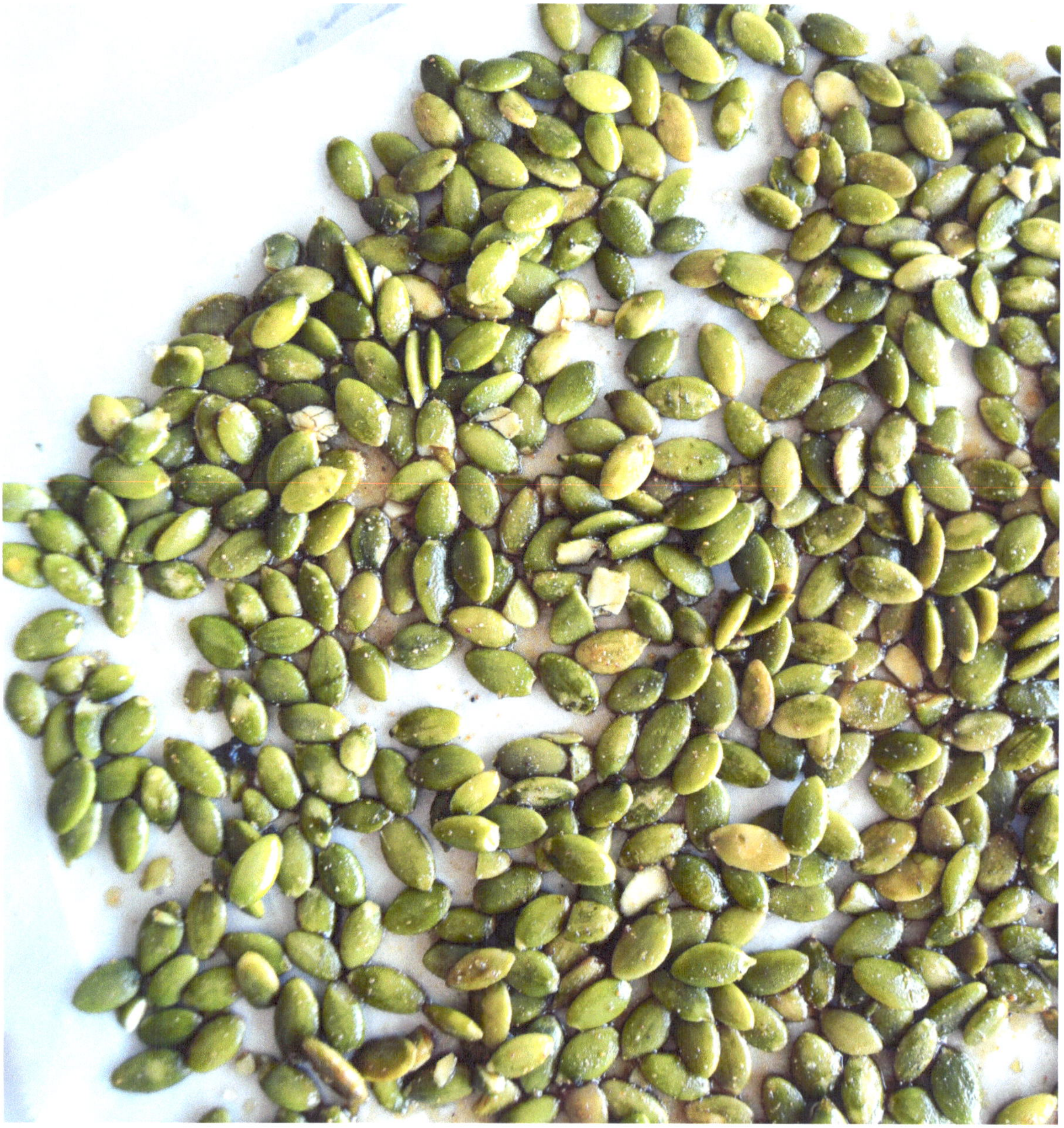

CANDIDED PEPITAS

Yield: 100 g

Ingredients

100 g raw pumpkin seeds (pepitas)
2 tbsp maple syrup
1/4 tsp licorice salt (from Saltverk)
1/2 tbsp ground ginger

Soak the pumpkin seeds in water for 4 hours. Drain well and put in a bowl.

Add all remaining ingredients into the bowl. Toss together.

Spread mixture over the dehydrator tray lined parchment paper or silicon paper.

Dehydrate at 42°C overnight or until completely dried and crispy.

WHITE CHOCOLATE

Ingredients

1/4 cup raw cacao butter melted
1/4 cup cashews soaked overnight
1 tbsp cashew butter
1 tsp lecithin powder
1/4 cup monk fruit powder
1/4 tsp licorice salt

Place the melted cacao butter, cashew butter and lecithin to Blendtec Twister jar. Blend until smooth. Then add the salt, monk fruit powder, cashews and blend again until completely smooth.

Pour the mixture thinly in a tray lined parchment paper. Top with desired dried fruits and nuts of your choice.

Freeze. Once done, break into shards and enjoy!

PEACH PUDDING

Ingredients

1 cup young coconut meat
1/2 cup cashews soaked
1 cup chopped peach
1/2 cup water
1/4 cup maple syrup
1 tsp vanilla bean powder
A pinch salt

Place all the ingredients in a high speed blender.

Blend until everything smooth and well combined.

Divide between bowls.

Chill overnight and serve with peach slices if desired.

GINGER LIME CHEESECAKE

Yield: 8-10 small bowls

Cheesecake
2 cups macadamia soaked
1/2 cup coconut oil
1/2 cup water
1/4 cup maple
1 tbsp nutritional yeast
1/2 cup lime juice
2 tbsp lime zest
A pinch salt

Ginger Hemp Crumble
2 cups hemp hearts
1 cup coconut flour
1/4 cup maple syrup
5-6 tbsp coconut milk
1 tbsp freshly grated ginger
1 tbsp cinnamon
1 tsp licorice salt

Except coconut oil, add all the ingredients in a high speed blender, blend until smooth.

Then add the coconut oil and blend to combine. Pour in the desired cake tin. Chill overnight.

To make ginger crumble, mix all ingredients in the food processor.
Evenly spread over the dehydrator sheet. Dehydrate at 42°C for 18-20 hours or overnight.

Once your cake is done, remove from the tin. Serve with ginger hemp crumbs on top.

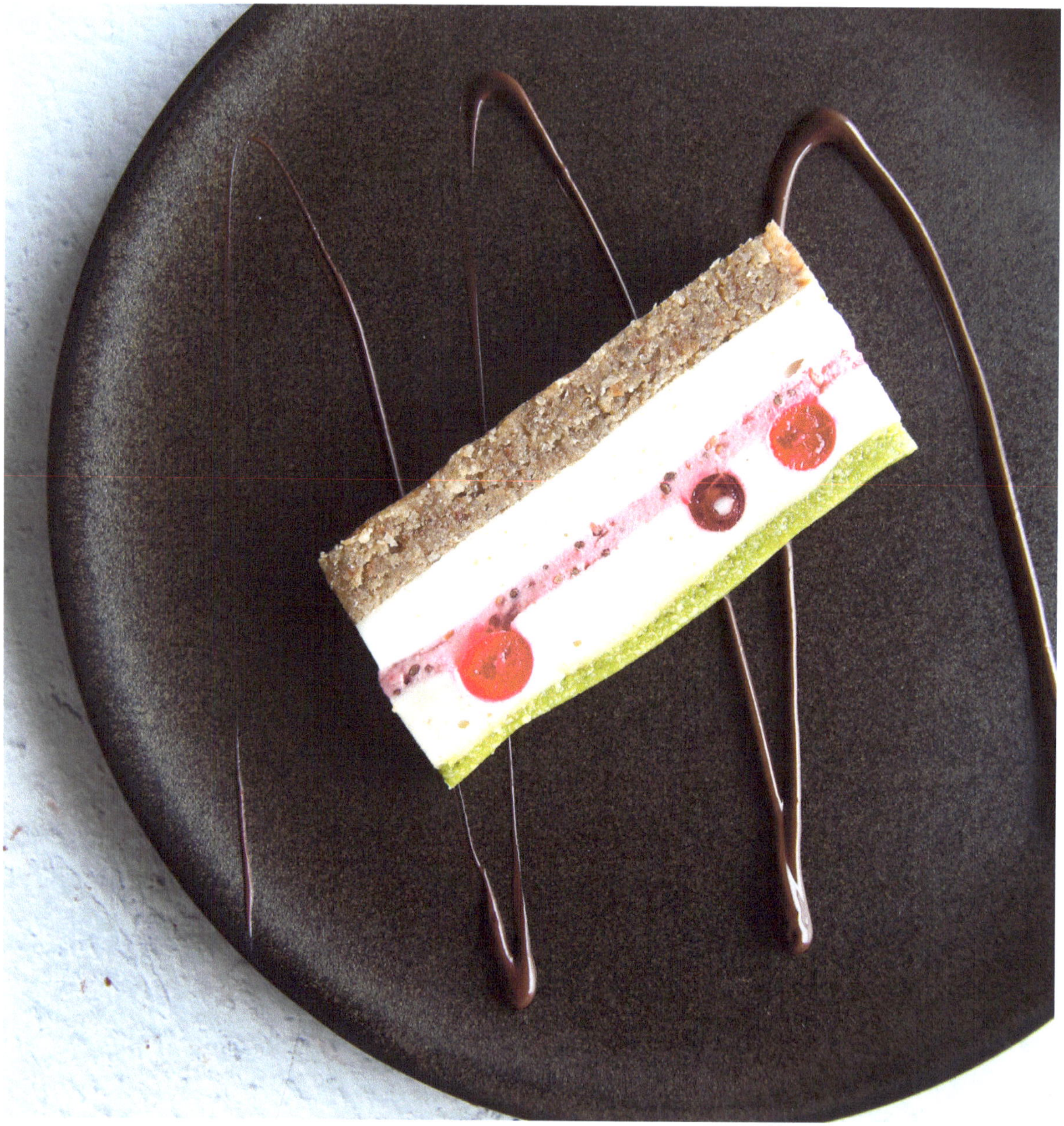

SWEDISH PRINCESS CAKE

Yield: 15 cm round cake

BASE

90 g almond flour
100 g date paste
35 g coconut flour
1 tbsp coconut oil
1/2 tsp vanilla extract

WHITE CREAM LAYER

160 g raw cashews soaked
3 tbsp maple syrup
3 tbsp lemon juice
40 g coconut oil melted
25 g raw cacao butter melted
100 g coconut cream

JAM LAYER

130 g raspberry chia jam (recipe on the lamingon cake page)
100 g white filling cream
15 g cacao butter melted

GREEN MARZIPAN LAYER

1 tsp matcha powder
90 g almond flour
4 tbsp maple syrup
20 g coconut flour
1/4 tsp medicine flower almond extract

To make the base add the almonds to a food processor and blitz until they are finely ground. Add the remaining ingredients for the base and continue to blitz until all the ingredients are broken down into a crumb. The mixture should press together like a dough between your fingers. Press the dough into the bottom of your cake tin. Pack it down firmly and set aside while you making filling.

To prepare the filling, add the cashews, coconut cream, maple syrup, lemon juice to your blender. Blend until they are smooth. Lastly add in the melted coconut oil, and coconut butter then blend further for 30 seconds to incorporate the oil into the mixture. Take around 100 gram of the cream and set aside to use it in mid layer later.
Pour half of the remaining cream over the cake crust. Place in the freezer to set for 20 minutes to set in order to prevent mixed layers.

Make raspberry chia jam according to raw jam recipe in this book. Place in a bowl, add 100 gram of the filling cream and melted cacao butter. Mix well in the bowl. Set aside.
Place almond and coconut flour into food processor, combine well. Then add maple syrup, almond extract and matcha. Mix until you get sticky dough.
When first cream layer is done, remove from the freeezer, add raspberry layer over the cashew filling, then set in the freezer next 25 minutes. Then pour remaining cashew filling. Freeze for 45 minutes. Remove cake from the mold. Cover with princess layer (green marzipan). Keep in the refrigerator for next 30 minutes before cutting and serve.

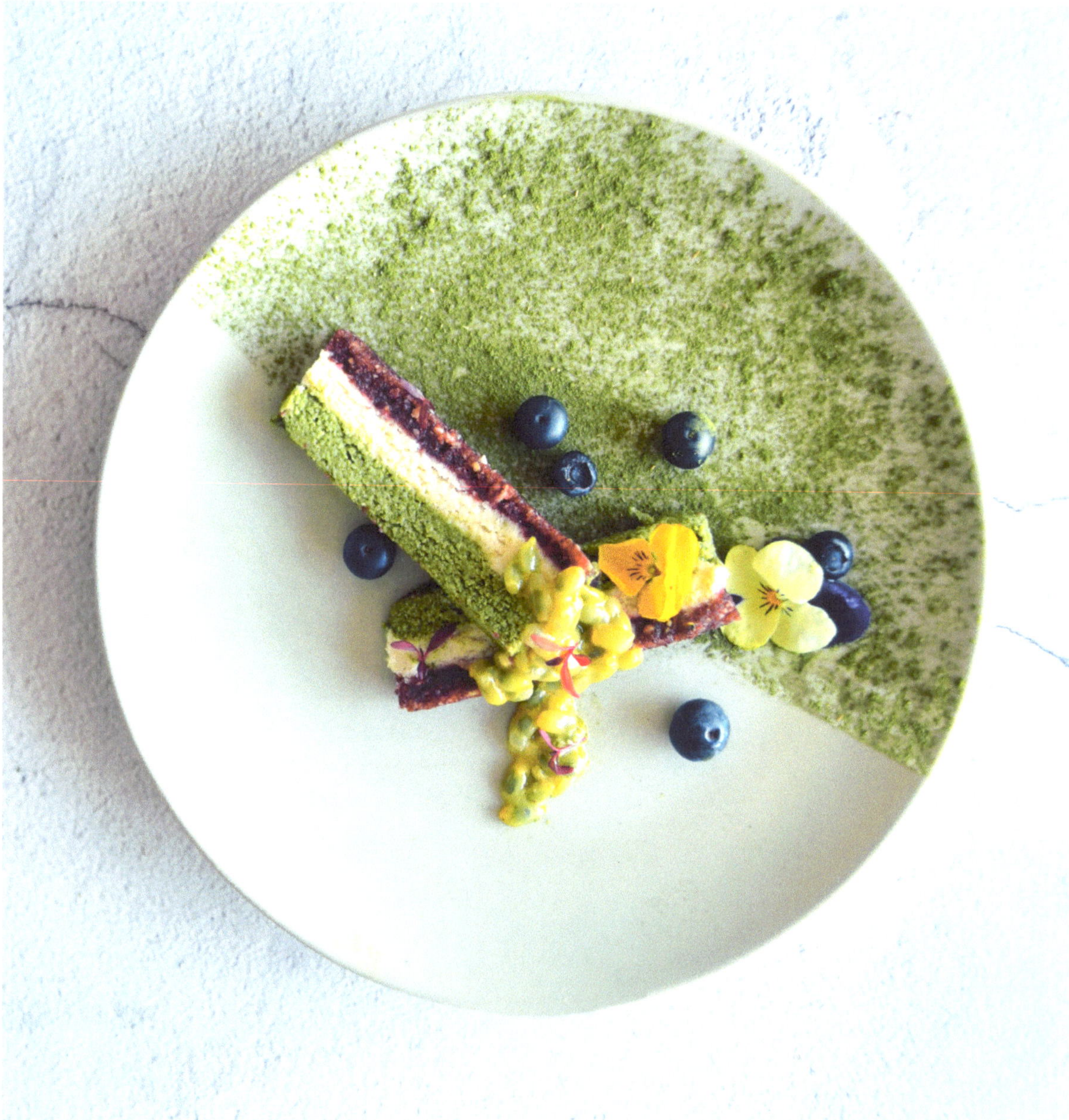

MATCHA BEETROOT CAKE

Yield: 15 cm round cake

Beet Layer

100 g almond meal
50 g coconut oil
105 g medjool dates
2 tbsp beetroot powder
1/4 licorice salt

White Layer

100 g coconut cream
130 g raw cashews soaked
2 tbsp maple syrup
2 tbsp coconut oil
1 tsp vanilla extract
3 tbsp lemon juice

Matcha Layer

2 tsp matcha powder
100 g raw cashews soaked
2 tbsp maple syrup
2 tbsp coconut oil
2 tbsp lemon juice
1 tsp vanilla extrach
A pinch of salt

Process all the beet layer ingredients in your food processor until sticky. Press the mixture into cake tin and place in the freezer to set while you work with your white and matcha layers.

In a food processor, process all white layer ingredients until smooth. Spread the mixture evenly over the beet layer, return to the freezer.
Once it has hardened. Process matcha layer until smooth, spread mixture over the white cream layer.

Back in freezer. After 2 hours, remove from the freezer. Cut into small long pieces. Take a blank paper , cover the half of plate, using a small tea-strainer, dust some matcha powder over the plate. Remove the paper. Place cake pieces on the plate. Decorate with fresh blueberry, passion fruit and edible flowers if desired. Enjoy!

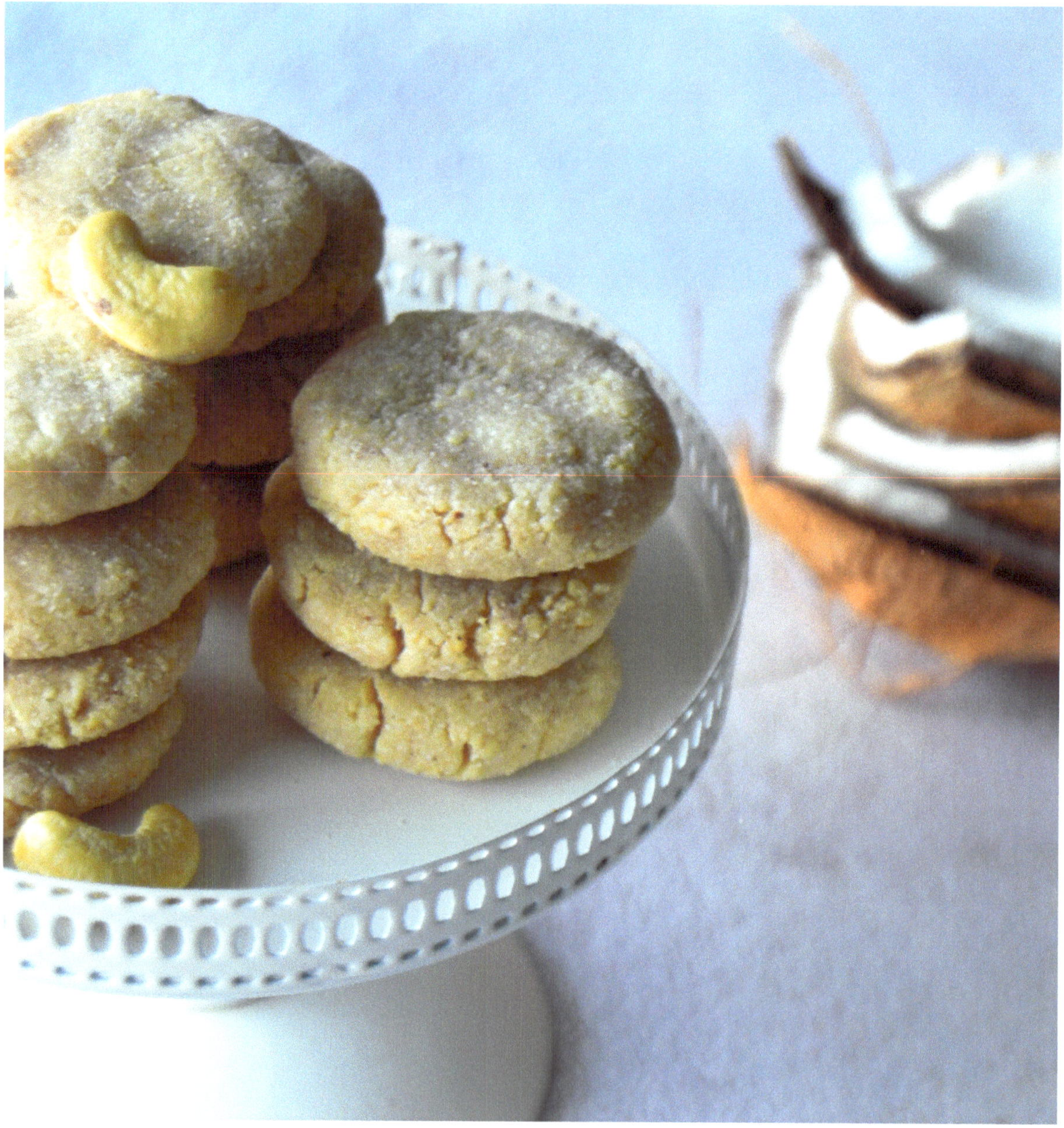

COCONUT CASHEW COOKIES

Yield: 12- 14 cookies

Ingredients

200 g raw cashews
300 g raw coconut flour
5-6 tbsp fresh coconut water
7 g psyllium husk powder
1 lemon juice,
1 tbsp maple syrup
1/2 tsp cinnamon
1/4 tsp nutmeg
1/4 tsp cardamom

Process the cashews in a food processor until they resemble course flour.

Add the coconut flour and process again until very well mixed. Add the lemon juice, psyllium husk powder, coconut water, maple and spices, mix again until combined well. (if it is a bit too wet add more coconut flour or if it is a bit dry add a tiny bit of coconut water.)

Shape into cookies. Dehydrate in the dehydrator for 5-6 hours at 42°C.

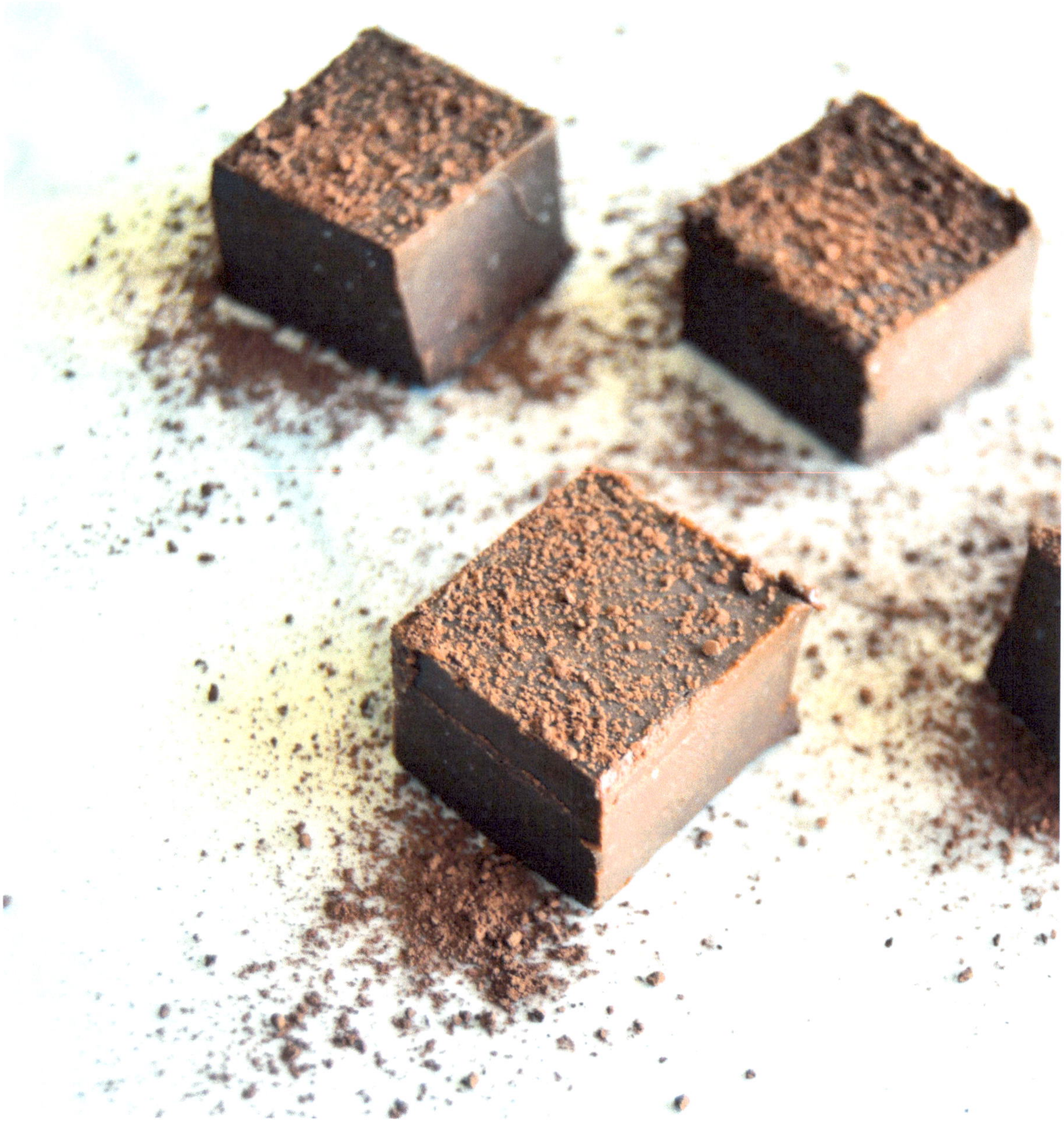

CHOCOLATE PUDGE

Yield: 4-6 person

Ingredients

100 g raw cacao paste melted
80 g coconut oil melted
50 g maple syrup
1 tsp coconut aminos
1 tsp vanilla bean powder
1/4 tsp licorice salt

Place the melted raw cacao paste and coconut oil in a bowl and stir to combine well.

Then add the maple syrup, coconut aminos, vanilla bean and licorice salt. Whisk well for couple of minutes until everything well combined.

In this step you may want to add some chopped almonds or hazelnuts if you want, otherwise it will still work.

Pour the mixture into square or preferred moulds and pop in the refrigerator to set for 20-30 minutes.

Once firmed up, pop them out of the mould and serve.

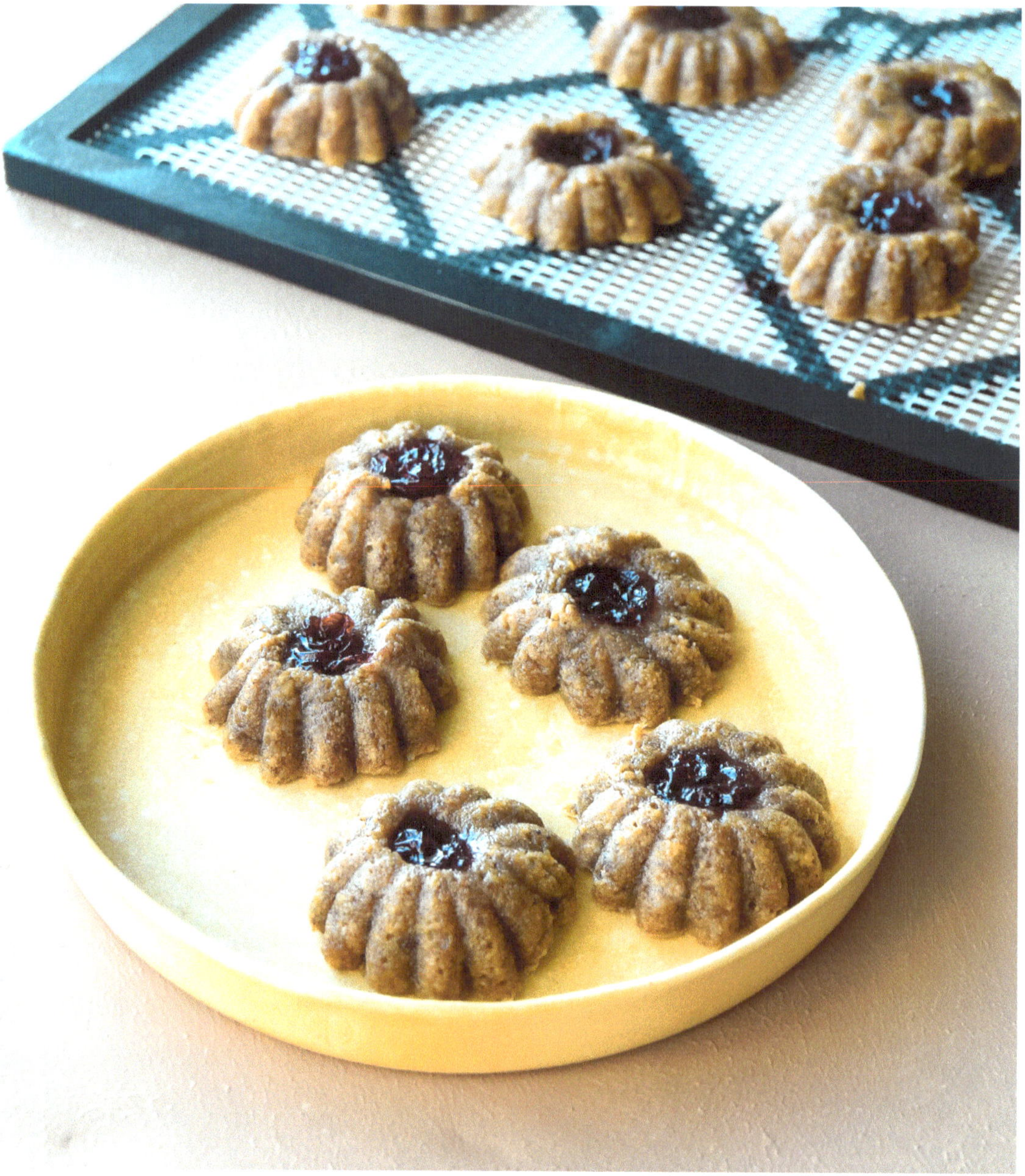

DEHYDRATED RAW COOKIES WITH LINGON JAM

Yield: 10-12 cookies

Cookies

1 tsp chia seeds + 2 tbsp water
1/2 cup sprouted oat flour
1 tsp cinnamon powder
1/2 tbsp raw coconut sugar
2 tbsp maple syrup
2 tbsp unroasted almond butter
1 tsp extra virgin olive oil
1/4 tsp salt
1/4 tsp baking soda

Jam

1/2 cup lingonberries
2 tbsp maple syrup
1 tbsp lemon juice
2 tbsp chia seeds

In a mixing bowl, mix chia seeds and water. Keep stirring for the first minute or so to prevent the chia seeds from clumping together. Then set asid for 5 minutes.
Then add the rest of ingredients in the chia seed mixture. Stir well to combine.
Transfer the dough onto a baking tray lined parchment paper. Lightly wet your hands with a little bit olive oil and shape the dough into small cookies, create small holes in the middle of the cookies with your fingers. I used a special mold from Pufz.se for these, if you don't have similar one, you can shape them with your hands.
The cookie won't spread, so shape it the way you want the end result to look like.
Dehydrate for 8 hours (or overnight)
Place all the jam ingredients in the blender, blend until smooth, set in the refrigerator for 2 hours.
After 8 hours, fill the holes of the cookies with lingonberry jam. Continue to dehydrate until fully dried both sides of the cookies in the Excalibur dehydrator.
It can be stored in the airtight container or jar up to 2 months. Once opened the jar, consume immediately for the best taste.

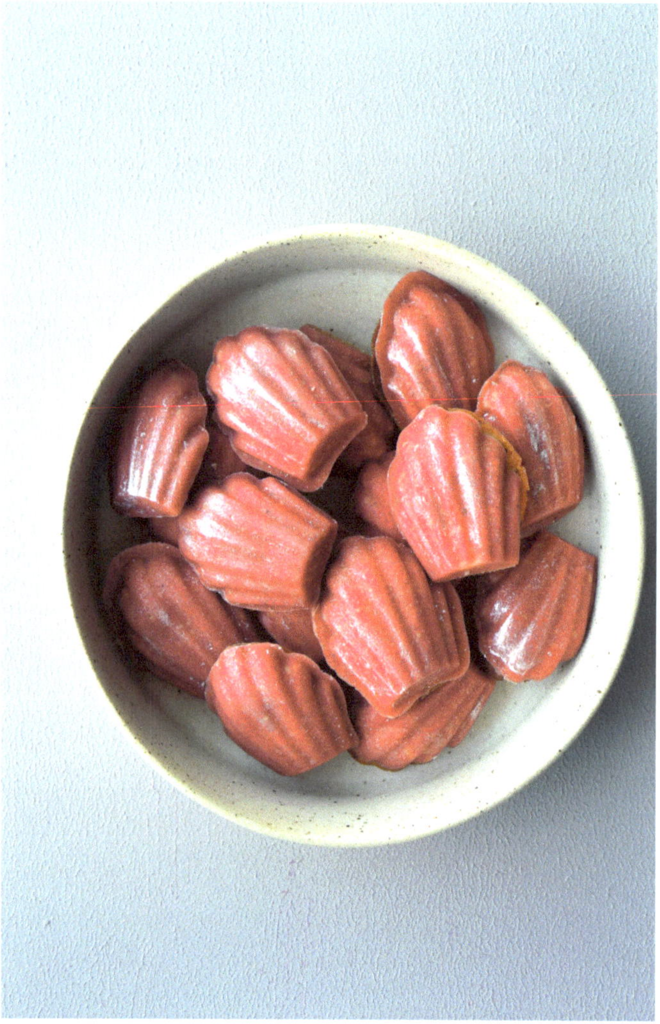

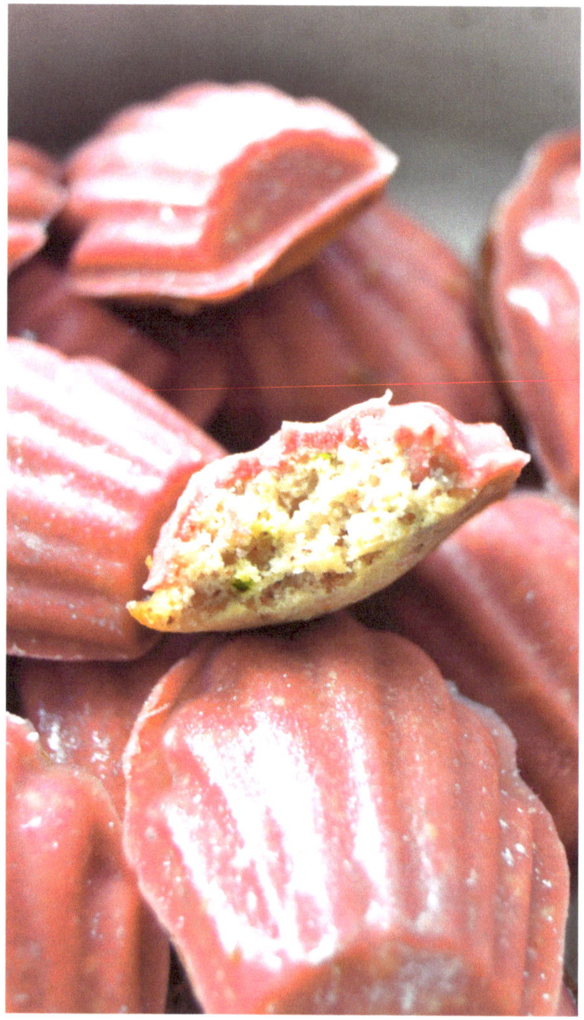

MINI MADELEINES

Yield: 16-18 pieces

Ingredients

120 g sprouted brown rice flour
50 g blanched almond flour
5 tbsp maple syrup
3 tbsp extra virgin olive oil
100 ml plant milk
1 tsp finely chopped lime zest
1/2 tsp baking soda
A pinch of salt

Strawberry Chocolate Shell

2 tbsp maple
50 g raw cacao butter
45 g hazelnut butter
4 tbsp freeze dried strawberry powder
1/4 tsp maca powder (optional)
A pinch of salt

This chocolate shell recipe is to make pink chocolate with berry flavour from scratch, alternatively you can also use a good tempered raw dark chocolate

In a large mixing bowl, whisk together the sprouted brown rice flour, blanched almond flour, maple, baking soda, and salt.
Then add the maple, plant milk and olive oil. Cover the bowl and refrigerate for 15-20 minutes.
Once refrigerated, transfer mixture in a pipping bag. Pipe the cold batter into each cavity, to the 3/4. You can also fill with the help of a teaspoon. Transfer the filled madeleine mould to the freezer for 10 minutes.
Place Madeleine mould into food dehydrator. (We use Excalibur) Start dehydrating at46°C for 2-3 hours, then flip the mould on the dehydrator sheet. Remove the mould. Then continue to dehydrate for 4-5 hours or overnight until completely dried.
Once madeleines are done, it is time to make chocolate shell. Using bain marie method and temperature control, melt the raw cacao butter maximum at46°C. Once melted, add the rest of the ingredients. Whisk well. Fill the each cavity to the 2/4, use a spoon to spread it. Top with your madeleine and slightly press it down. Repeat with the remaining chocolate and madeleines and place the Madeleine mould in the freezer for about 15 minutes or until the chocolate has hardened and easy to remove the madeleines.

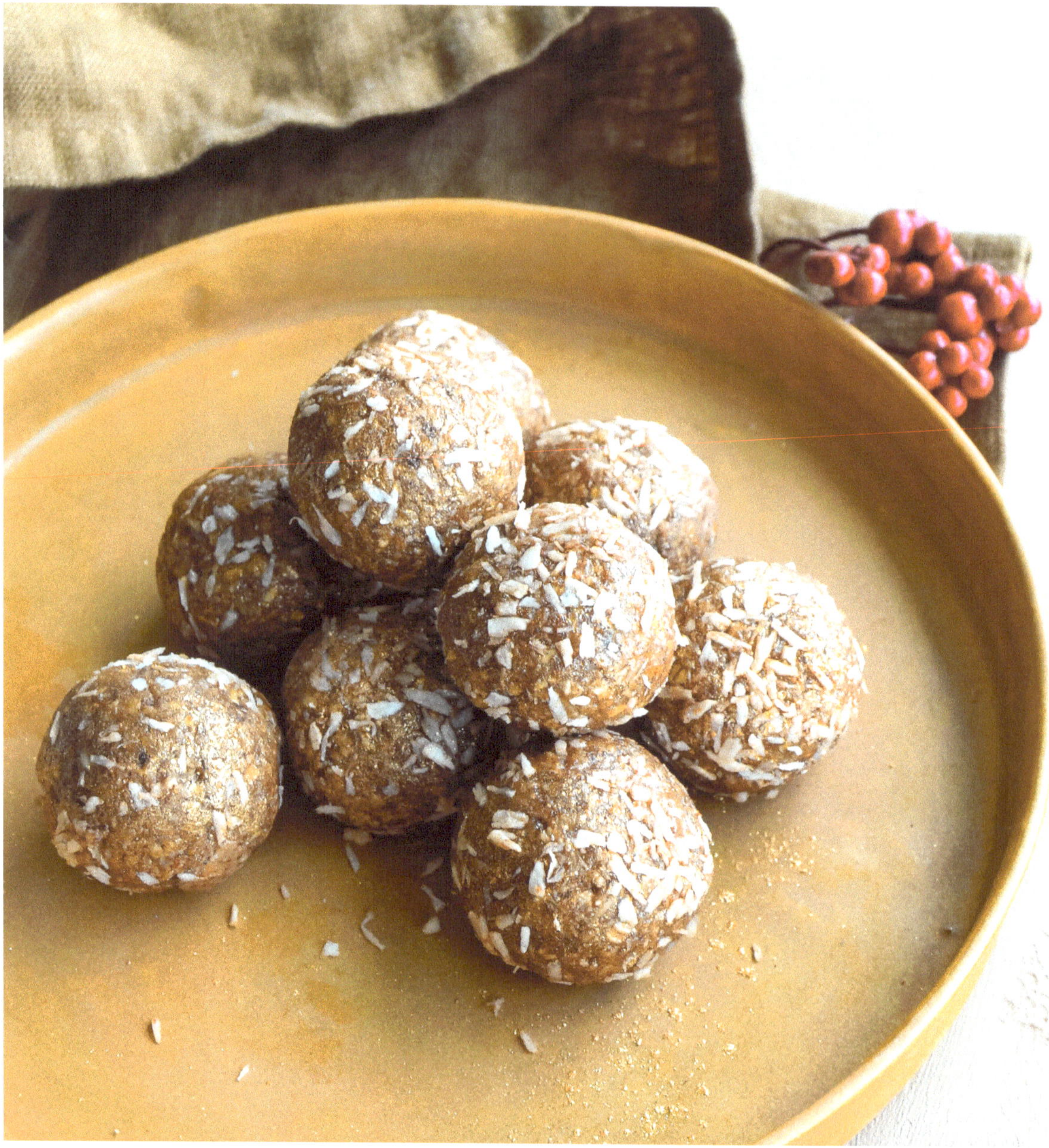

GINGERBREAD BALLS

Yield: 8-10 balls

Ingredients

130 g sprouted rolled oat flour
65 g desiccated coconut
3 tbsp almond butter
2 tbsp maple syrup (or agave, coconut nectar syrup, date syrup etc)
1 tbsp fresh orange juice
1/2 tsp cinnamon
1/8 tsp ginger
1/8 tsp cardamom
A pinch nutmeg

Filling

2 tbsp almond butter
1 tbsp maple syrup

For garnish

4 tbsp desiccated coconut
1 tsp gold powder
1/ tsp cinnamon powder

Place all the ingredients in a food processor. Blend until you get a smooth sticky dough.
Using your hands make small balls.
In a small bowl, mix maple and almond butter. Pour into syringe. Then squeeze into the balls.
Cover them in desiccated coconut cinnamon gold powder mix. Enjoy!

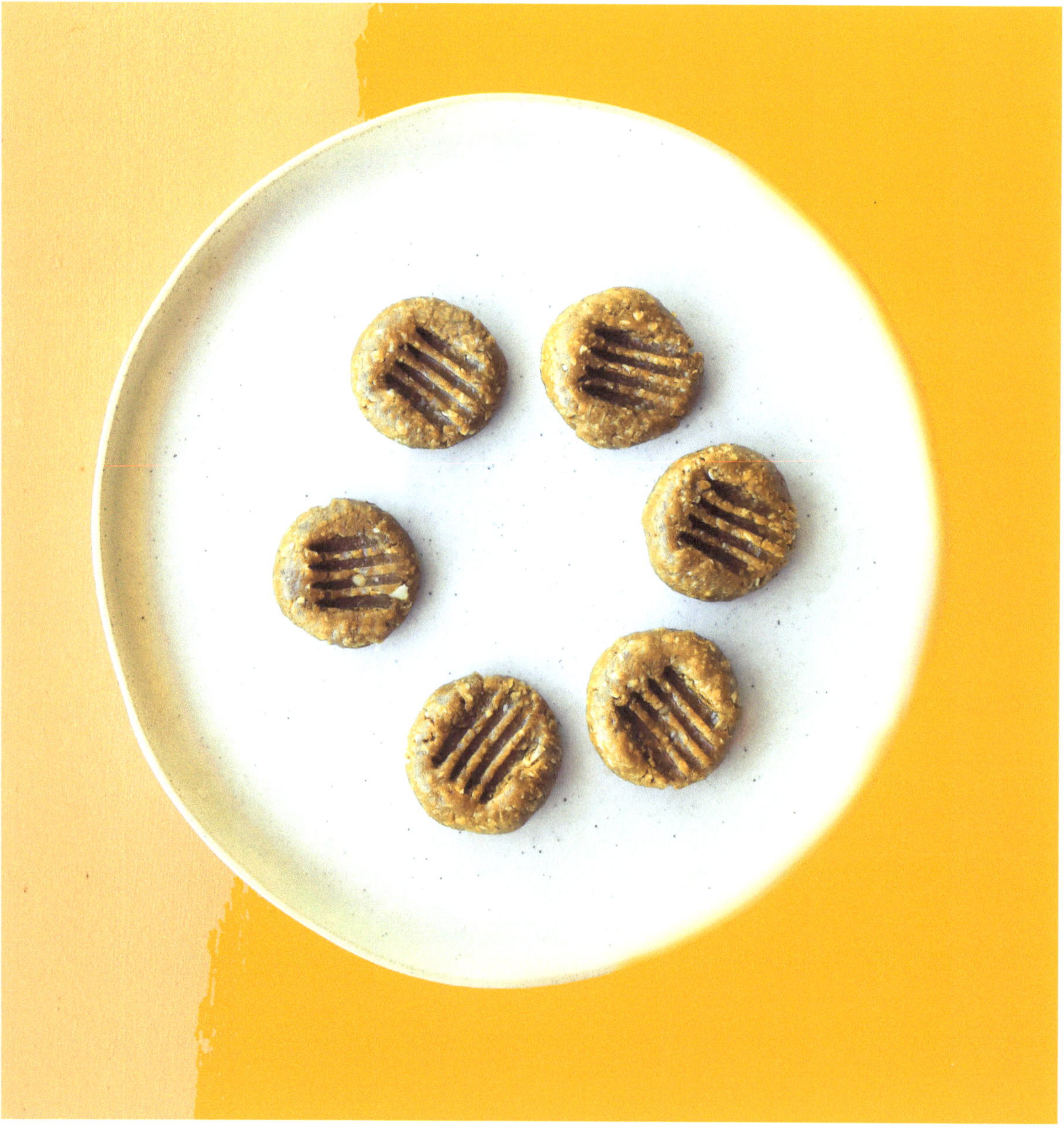

ALMOND BUTTER COOKIES

Yield: 12-14 pieces

Ingredients

95 g gluten-free sprouted oat flour
25 g maca or carob powder
90 g maple syrup
180 g raw almond butter
1/2 tsp salt

Place the sprouted oat flour, maca powder and salt in a high speed food processor, blend until combined well.

Add the almoond butter and maple, process to combine. You will get a nice smooth sticky dough. It can be easily shape. If it is too wet, add a little bit more oat flour, one tablespoon at a time.

Remove the dough from the food processor.
Make small balls with your hands. Put on the parchment paper.

Using the back of the fork, press down the cookies to shape.
Set in the refrigerator for 2 hours before serving.

"YOU ALREADY KNOW EVERYTHING, RAW FOOD IS JUST A TOOL TO SIMPLY MAKES YOU AWARE OF IT!"

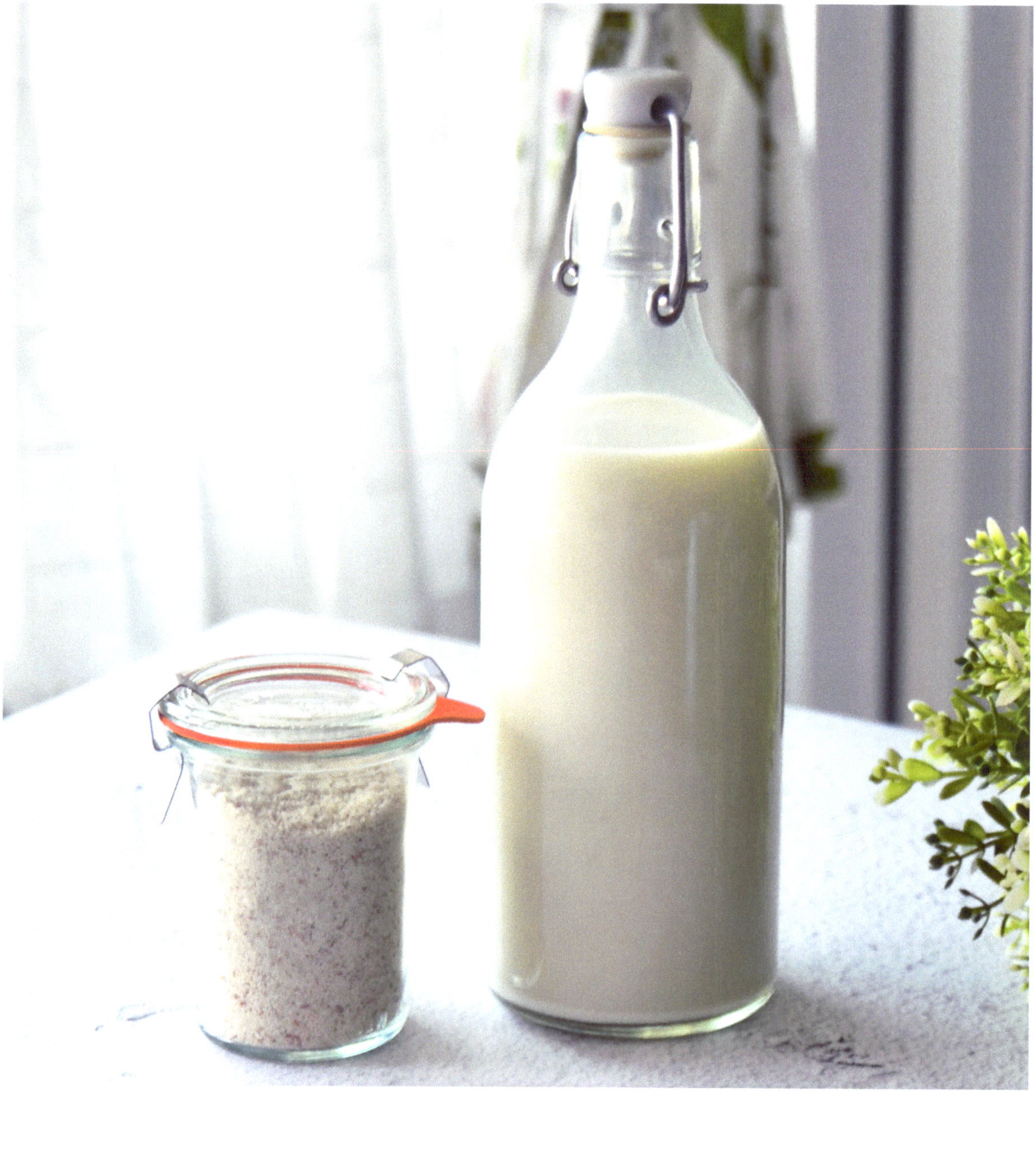

SESAME MILK

Yield: 750 ml

Ingredients

1 cup white sesame
3 cups filtered water
1 tsp vanilla extract
2 tbsp maple syrup
A pinch cardamom
A pinch licorice salt

Instructions

Place sesame seeds and water into your blender, mix on high speed for 2-3 minutes.

Using a nut milk bag, strain your milk. Rinse your blender, and pour the strained milk back in.

Add the maple syrup, vanilla, and salt, and process on low for just a few seconds to combine.

Store the milk in a sealed container in the fridge. Sesame milk will keep for about 3 days in a very cold fridge.

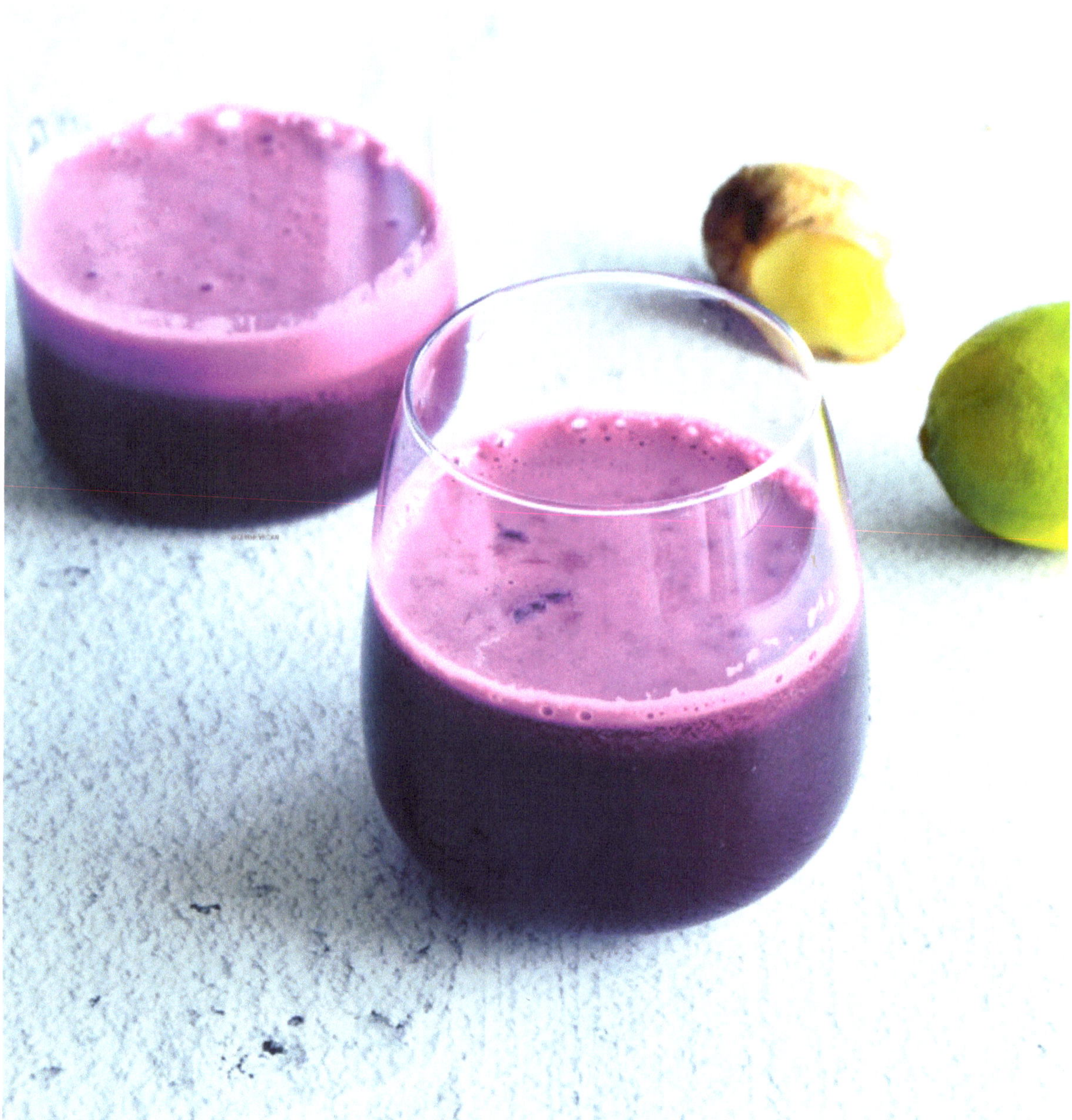

JUICES

Some delicious juice combinations you will find below. You can use a slow juicer or regular one to juice the fruits and vegetables. Make sure you washed and peeled well.

BEET CELERY

4 celery stalks
2 green apples
1 medium carrot
1 medium beetroo

CABBAGE MAJORAM

1/2 head purple cabbage
1 red apple
2 cucumber
1 inch ginger
2-3 majoram springs
1 lemon

SPINACH CARROT

1 small radish
1 celery stalk
1 cup baby spinach
6 small carrots
2 large tomatoes

CAYENNE CELERY

1 celery stalk
1 red bell pepper
A pinch cayenne
3 tomatoes

KALE PINEAPPLE

4 kale leaves
8 carrots
1 large pineapple
20 g basil
7 g fresh ginger

FENNEL APPLE

1/4 pomelo
3 granny smith apple
1/2 fennel bulb
1 -2 beetroot leaves

DETOX MIXTURE

5 celery stalks
1 zucchini
A handful collard greens
2 granny smith apple

RASPBERRY MINT

2 cups raspberries
1 cup blackberries
1 lime
20 g fresh mint

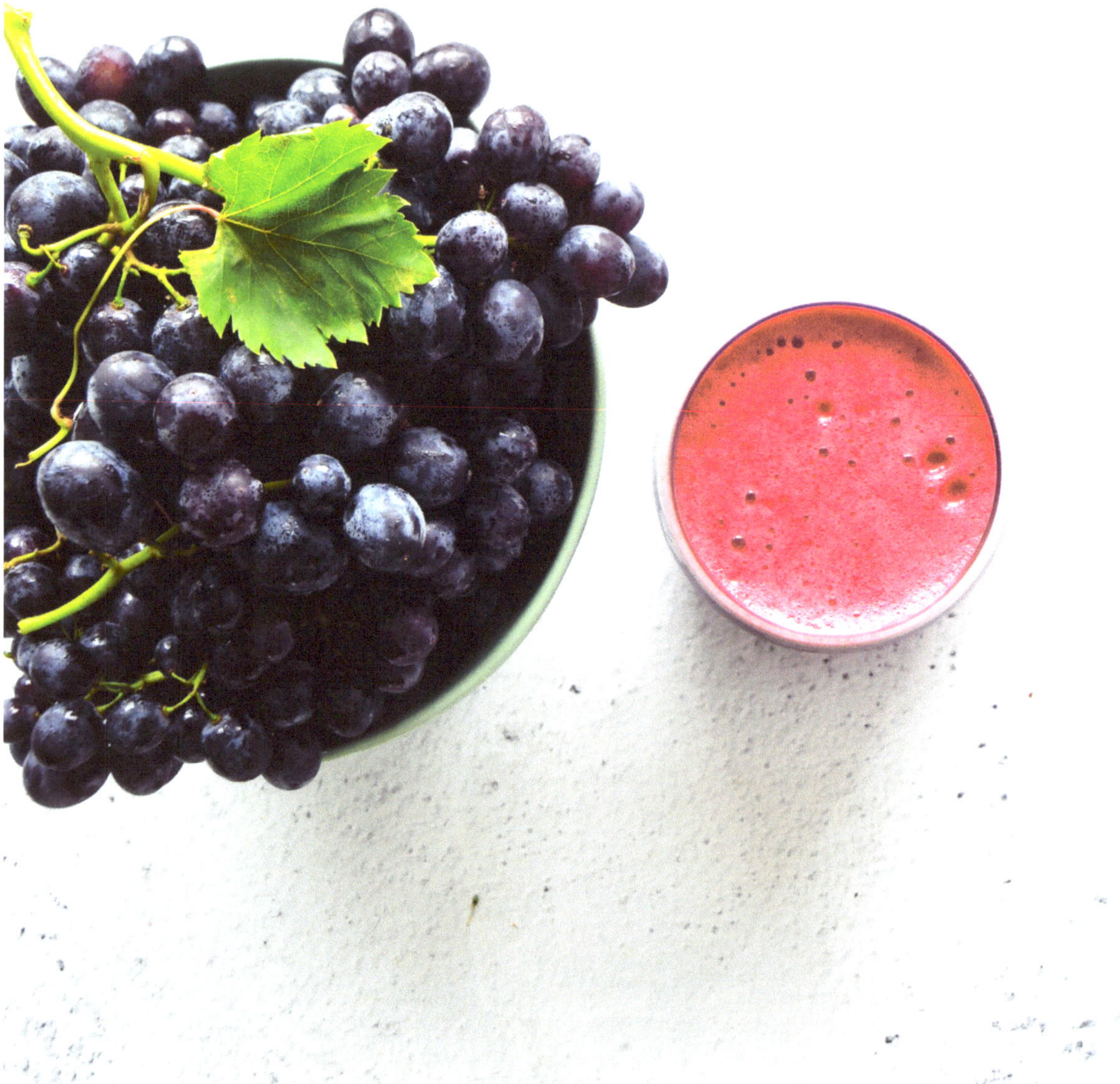

TAKE ENZYMES WITH JUICE

There are thounsands of toxins in the environment today. Juicing not only helps to body to dispose of these toxins but also provides it with necessary enxymes. But it is very important to choose only organic fruits and veggies to help in removal of toxins. Enzymes may be the key in preventing chronical diaeses and extending our lifespan. As we age, we produce fewer enzymes necessary for healthy digestion. It is impossible for our bodies to properly break down food without these enzymes.

Fresh juice helps us to get enough enzymes that come from raw vegetables, greens and fruits. Just about anyone eats a cooked diet. Enzymes are destroyed when a food is cooked, microwaved, pasteurized, processed, canned, packaged or genetically engineered.
We need enyzmes for every chemical action. Our all cells, organs, bones because of enyzmes. Everything depends on enyzmes includingr immune and digestive system, bloodstream, kidneys, liver and much more. Vitamins, minearls or hormones can not do any work without enzymes. Even our ability to feel, think and breathe are dependening on enzymes.

We need enzymes for proper digestion health, antiaging and cell repair. If you have weak nails, thin hair, dull skin, insomnia, mood swings, or fatigue it is likely you are not properly digesting your food.
Raw food is not a new concept, scientists discovered the importance of enzymes contained in only raw foods. Bad dietary and lifestyle habits, including consumption of sugar, fats, white flour, cooked and processed food, too much stress and being exposed to environmental pollution might all contribute to enzyme deficiency.
So what is the soluiton?
We should juice raw organic vegetables and fruits everyday. They will supply our body with needed enyzmes.

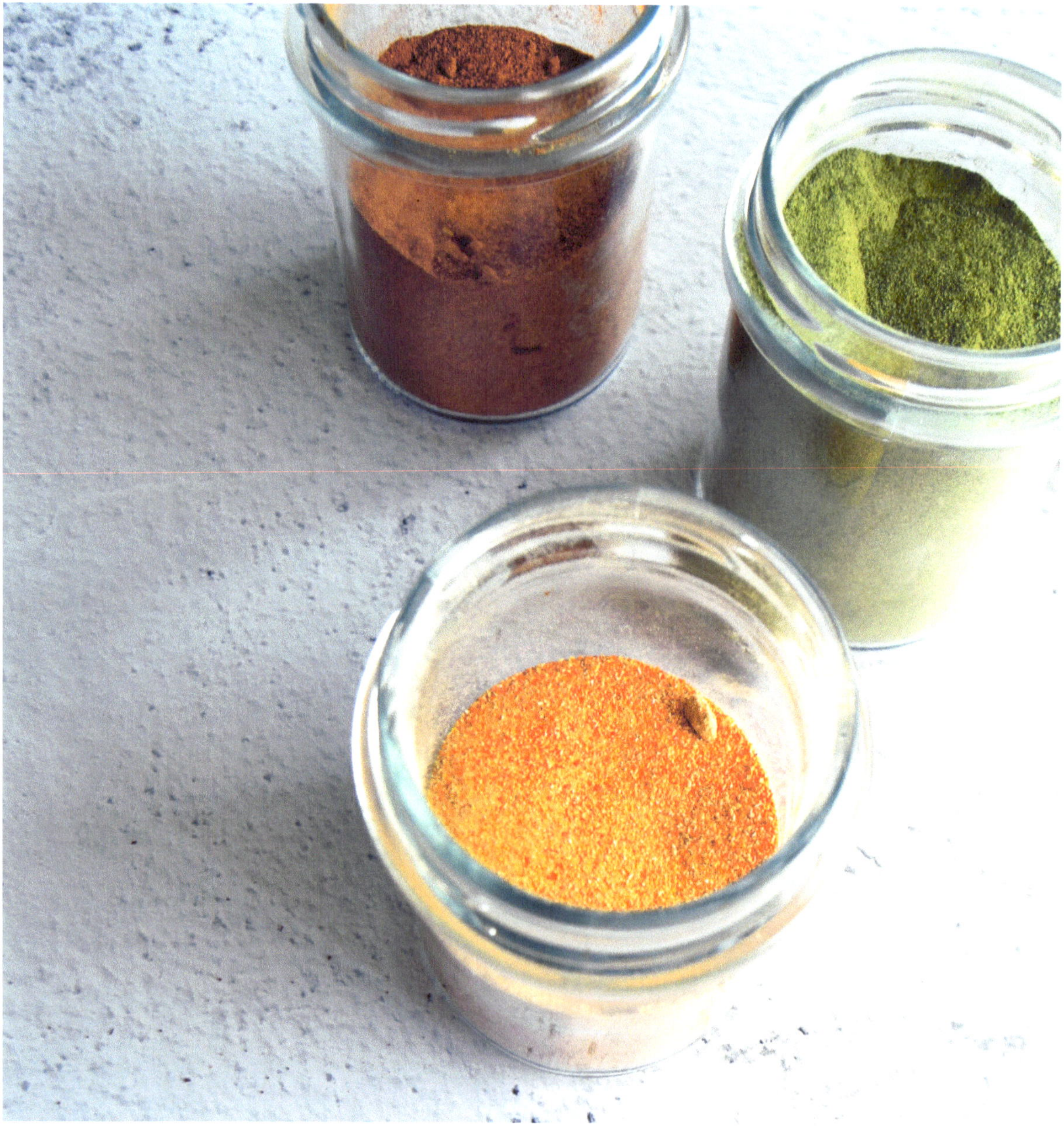

JUICE PULP POWDER

Spread the juice pulp evenly over dehydrator sheets, set your dehydrator at 115° F and dehydrate until completely dried. It usually takes between 4 to 8 hours, depending on the moisture of your home, the moisture content of your juice pulp and your dehydrator.

When it is dried, just throw the dry juice pulp in a high speed blender (just make sure they're fully cool first) give it several quick pulses, keep stopping it to allow the pulp pieces to settle.
Then move to blend, make sure if you get any bigger pieces that have not powdered well throw them back into the blender. Pour through a mesh strainer (this helps keep out the larger pieces) into a jar. If you want this stuff pretty powdery, then use a coffee grinder to create an ultra fine powder. Store in cool, dark and dry place.

Use frozen fruit or vegetable pulp to add flavor, texture, and moisture to muffins, cakes. Add to juice pulp to raw breads, use vegetable pulp to make super healthy raw wraps, flatbreads, crackers.

Use in homemade sauces, dips, spreads, dressings. Add to your favorite veggie burgers, pizza crust. Add to a soups or smoothies to thicken and boost fiber. Make juice pulp veggie stock, use it as a sprinkle on top of salads ... options are infinitive, have fun in the kitchen!

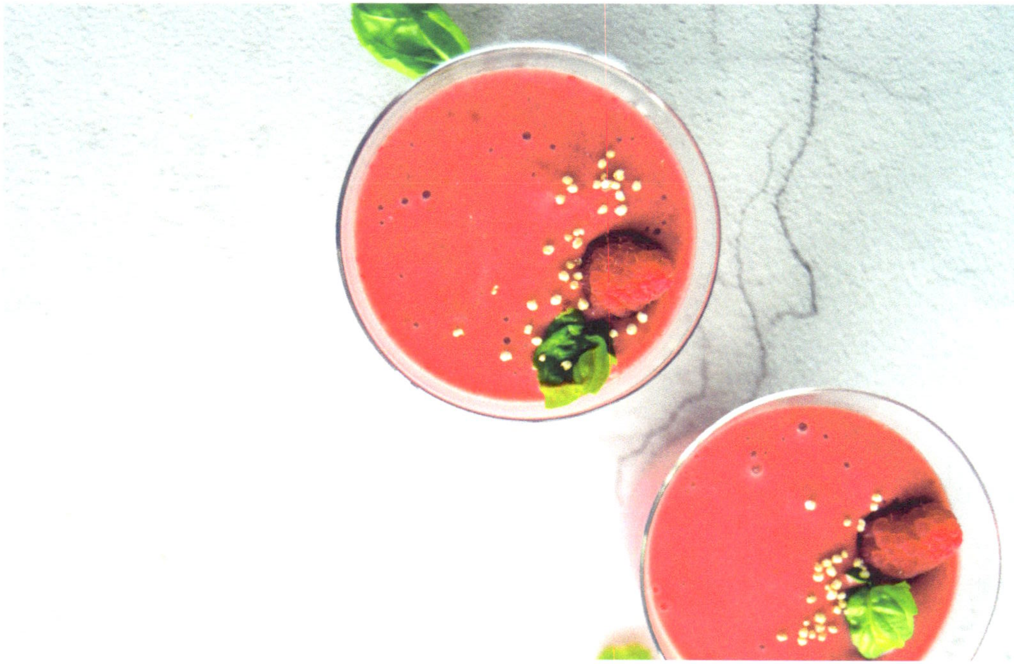

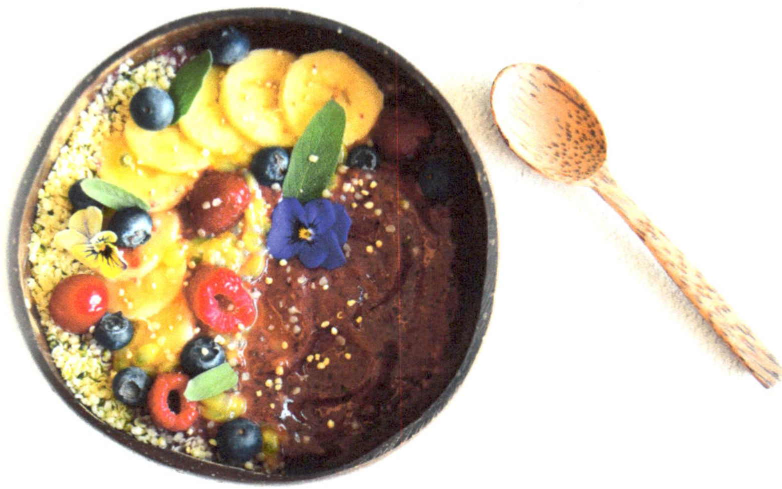

SMOOTHIES

Some delicious smoothie combinations you will find below. Place the ingredients to your blender, blend until smooth. Top with desired nuts, fruits and flowers. Enjoy!

ACAI BOWL

1 frozen banana
1 cup frozen acai puree
1/4 cup pineapple
1 cup frozen mixed berries
1 tbsp maple
1/4 cup almond milk
1/4 cup coconut yogurt

GREEN SMOOTHIE

1 cup sesame milk
1 cup fresh spinach
1 frozen banana
1/2 avocado

FOREST FRUITS SMOOTHIE

1 tbsp flaxseed
1/2 cup frozen bananas
1/2 cup frozen blackberries
1/2 cup frozen blueberries
1/2 cup frozen raspberries
1 cup coconut water

SUNSHINE SMOOTHIE

1/4 cup sprouted rolled oats
1/2 cup frozen mango
1 frozen banana
1/4 cup almond milk
1 tsp turmeric powder or freshly juiced
1 tsp ginger powder or fresh one grated

APPLE PIE SMOOTHIE

1 cup frozen bananas
1 red apple diced
2 tbsp almond butter
1/4 cup almond milk
2 soft dates
1/2 tsp cinnamon
1/4 tsp cardamom
A pinch salt

PUMPKIN PIE SMOOTHIE

1/4 cup shredded raw pumpkins
1 cup frozen bananas
1 cup almond milk
1/2 tsp cinnamon powder
1/4 cup dried raisins
A pinch salt

BEETROOT CHERRY SMOOTHIE

1/4 cup shredded beetroot
1 cup frozen bananas
1 cup almond milk
1/4 cup frozen cherries
A pinch salt

PINA COLADA SMOOTHIE

1/2 pineapple
1 cup frozen bananas
1 cup coconut water
1/2 tsp turmeric

index

A

B

C

D

E

F

G

H

I

J

K

L

M

T

U

W

Z

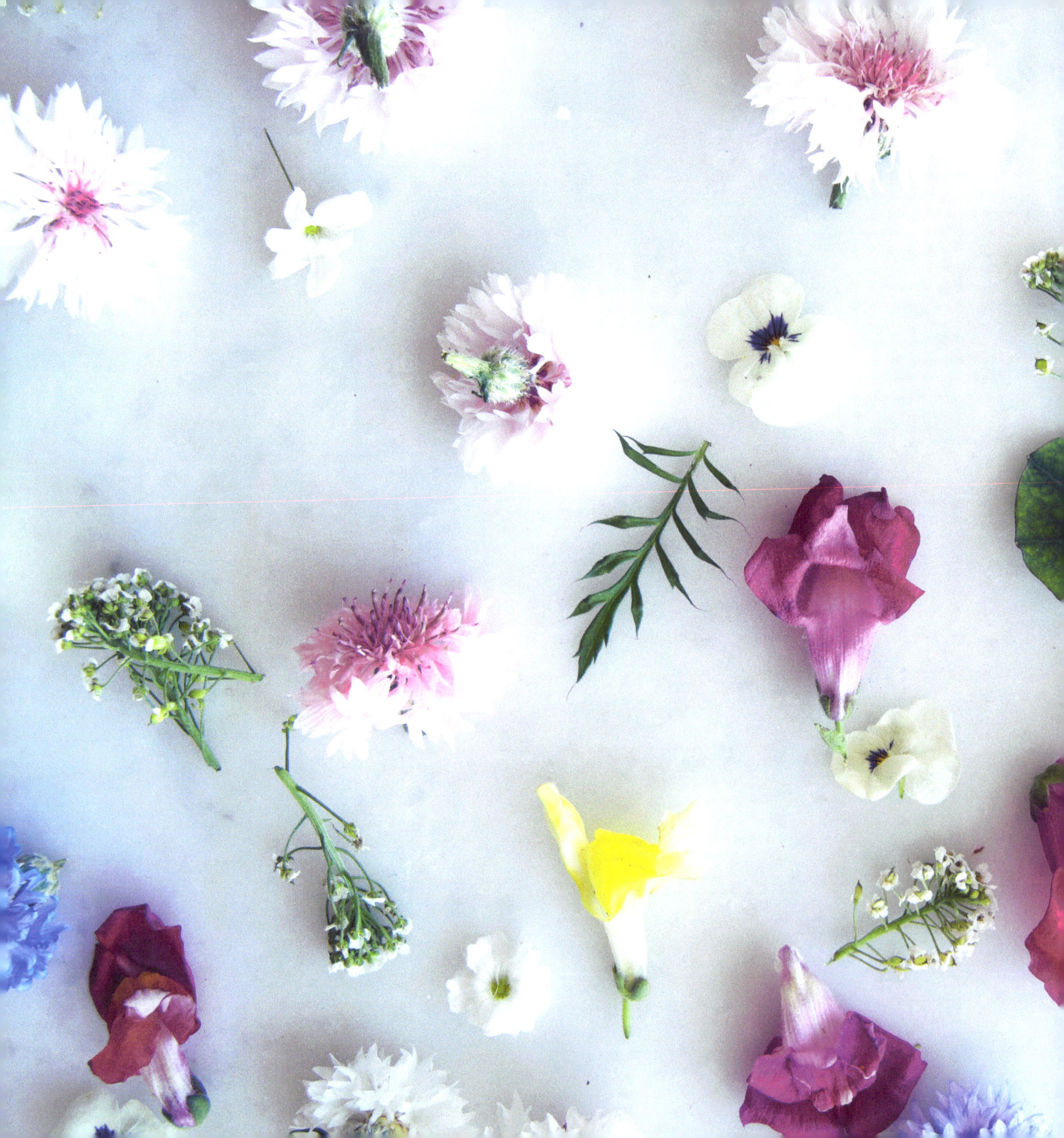

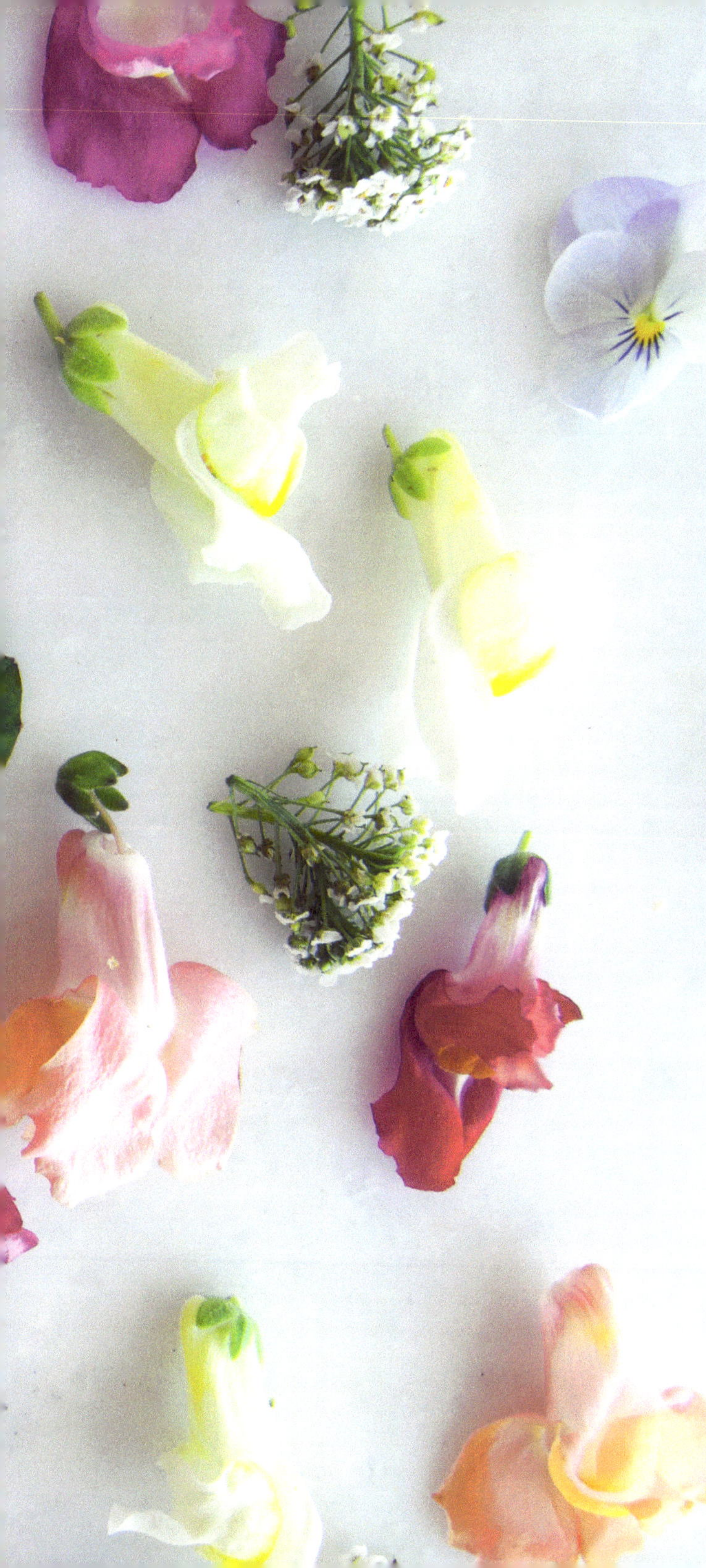

acknowledgments

This book was first written in 2018, published in 2019. The recipes have been tried by hundreds of people all over the world. I would like to thank you all, and express my great gratitude.
In 2022 we decided to expand, edit and redesign the book "Green & Awake: Gourmet Raw". We wanted to use the same design in this book as our much-loved and reader-friendly "Mad About Raw" book.
We found and fixed a few typos, added brand new recipes with the new photos. I hope you like this new edition as much as we do!

Nazlı Develi

about the author

Nazlı Develi is a plant food designer, an inventive, aesthetically minded hands-on chef and artist with an eye for details and the founder of GREEN & AWAKE: Plant Food Design Studio.

She specialized in wholesome plant-based and raw cuisine, restaurant consultancy, recipe development, workshops, chef training and creative concepts, all rooted in food expression with nature as a core.

Obsessed with art, design, health, wellness and experimental flavours, she's strongly committed to spreading awareness about plant-based food as the most sustainable and necessary alternative for the planet.

Instagram: @gurmevegan I @greenandawake
Website: www.gurmevegan.com
www.greenandawake.com

www.ingramcontent.com/pod-product-compliance
Lightning Source LLC
LaVergne TN
LVHW071238210926
848486LV00007B/295